Cultural Assessment in Clinical Psychiatry

Committee on Cultural Psychiatry

Ezra Griffith, M.D., *Chairperson*
Renato D. Alarcón, M.D., M.P.H., *Project Coordinator*
Irma Bland, M.D.
Prakash Desai, M.D.
Edward F. Foulks, M.D., Ph.D.
Frederick Jacobsen, M.D., M.P.H.
Roberto Lewis-Fernandez, M.D.
Francis Lu, M.D.
Maria Oquendo, M.D.
Pedro Ruiz, M.D.
J. Arturo Silva, M.D.
Ronald Wintrob, M.D.
Joe Yamamoto, M.D.
Trevia F. Hayden, M.D. (Fellow)
Robert L. Harvey, M.D. (Consultant)
J. Charles Ndlela, M.D., M.P.H. (Consultant)
Dora Wang, M.D. (Consultant)

Cultural Assessment in Clinical Psychiatry

Formulated by the
Committee on Cultural Psychiatry

Group for the Advancement of Psychiatry
Report No. 145

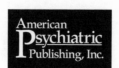

Washington, DC
London, England

Copyright © 2002 Group for the Advancement of Psychiatry
ALL RIGHTS RESERVED

Manufactured in the United States of America on acid-free paper
06 05 04 03 02   5 4 3 2 1
First Edition

American Psychiatric Publishing, Inc.
1400 K Street, N.W.
Washington, DC 20005
www.appi.org

Library of Congress Cataloging-in-Publication Data
Cultural assessment in clinical psychiatry / formulated by the Committee on Cultural Psychiatry, Group for the Advancement of Psychiatry.
     p. ; cm.—(Report ; no. 145)
Includes bibliographical references and index.
ISBN 0-87318-144-1 (alk. paper)
   1. Cultural psychiatry—United States. 2. Psychiatry, Transcultural. I. Group for the Advancement of Psychiatry. Committee on Cultural Psychiatry.
II. Report (Group for the Advancement of Psychiatry : 1984) ; no. 145.
   [DNLM: 1. Community Psychiatry. 2. Cross-Cultural Comparison.
3. Cultural Characteristics. 4. Cultural Diversity. WM 30.6 C9676 2001]
RC455.4.E8 C788 2001
616.89—dc21

                                2001027936

British Library Cataloguing in Publication Data
A CIP record is available from the British Library.

Contents

Introduction

Human beings reflect, in a complex set of everyday behaviors, the fact that they are repositories of a myriad of biological, social, psychological, and cultural influences. In the medical field, the doctor–patient relationship follows cultural rules as much as does the patient's attitude toward taking pills or undergoing procedures. The health care delivery system of the United States also faces the growth, as well as the economic and cultural needs, of ethnic minority groups in various parts of the country. Many professional organizations in mental health have acknowledged this reality and have provided practical tools for improving clinical services to these groups. Hence, in this volume is proposed a contemporary pragmatic understanding of how culture intertwines with and relates to mental health and mental illness. We offer this by considering specific cultural variables and applying DSM-IV-TR (American Psychiatric Association 2000) guidelines for use of the cultural formulation in a series of clinical case examples.

The first chapter presents a brief historical perspective of cultural psychiatry over the last several decades and defines five essential dimensions of cultural psychiatry as a clinical endeavor.

The second chapter includes a succinct but thorough description of the main cultural variables influencing clinical work. This list of variables, by no means exhaustive, emphasizes their conceptual connections and clinical relevance to the five essential dimensions of cultural psychiatry. The complexity of these variables—from gender, sexual orientation, and age to religious/spiritual beliefs, myths, traditions, folklore, and dietary habits and patterns—becomes greater as we move to consideration of socioeconomic status, cultural identity, country of origin, education, and language. The final set of variables involves racial and ethnic factors that, when taken together with the other elements, highlight the unique personal identity of each individual patient. The discussion of each variable centers on its roles and functions, both positive and negative, as they relate to health and illness behavior, expression of symptoms, explanatory models, stress causation, and social systems. Ultimately, each variable affects diagnosis and treatment outcomes.

The third chapter is a historical account and a detailed analysis of the cultural formulation presented in DSM-IV-TR (American Psychiatric Association 2000, Appendix I), the newest instrument for the thorough clinical assessment of any patient who comes to the professional's attention. Practical examples, as well as an analysis of the items included in each of the four specific areas of the cultural formulation, provide the reader with a useful tool for the cultural assessment of a variety of clinical events.

Perhaps the most important aspect of the book is the presentation in the fourth chapter of five cases reflecting a wide variety of clinical situations and the role of cultural factors in their causation, course, management, and outcome. These cases explore the previously mentioned cultural variables and follow the structure outlined by the *American Psychiatric Association Practice Guidelines for Psychiatric Evaluation of Adults* (American Psychiatric Association 1995). There is special emphasis on the application of the tenets of the cultural formulation appearing in DSM-IV (American Psychiatric Association 1994) and DSM-IV-TR. A pertinent literature review, as well as comments by the authors based on their specific expertise and clinical interests, completes each clinical discussion.

The fifth and final chapter summarizes the contributions made in previous sections and outlines conclusions and suggestions regarding the various issues raised by a thorough cultural assessment process in clinical psychiatry. The Group for the Advancement of Psychiatry (GAP) Committee on Cultural Psychiatry believes that this book meets a significant need of many psychiatrists and other mental health professionals committed to giving their patients the most comprehensive and qualitatively useful care possible. A solid cultural approach provides a valuable anchor for this process.

■ References

American Psychiatric Association: Diagnostic and Statistical Manual of Mental Disorders, 4th Edition. Washington, DC, American Psychiatric Association, 1994

American Psychiatric Association: Practice Guidelines for Psychiatric Evaluation of Adults. Washington, DC, American Psychiatric Association, 1995

American Psychiatric Association: Diagnostic and Statistical Manual of Mental Disorders, 4th Edition, Text Revision. Washington, DC, American Psychiatric Association, 2000

1

Culture in Clinical Psychiatry: History and Scope

In this chapter we succinctly review the main historical elements in cultural psychiatry's evolution, particularly during the last two decades. We also outline the theoretical background of what makes, or should make, culturally competent practitioners. Some essential definitions set the stage for an applied cultural psychiatry, systematized through five clinical dimensions and buttressed by relevant research.

The conventional clinical approach to psychiatric disorders emphasizes the basic precepts of Western medicine. This approach views the patient's illness as a collection of recognizable symptoms and signs codified by a predetermined diagnostic system. The study of such clinical manifestations evolves, in most cases, into the characterization of syndromes and, ultimately, into a nosological label. In turn, this process ideally guides the clinician through a set of procedures aimed at confirming the diagnostic impression and initiating a treatment plan (Cooper 1983). Although the diagnostic and therapeutic tools may be linked to the special nature of the symptoms, this sequence follows essentially the disease model—that is, etiological agents working their pathological ways in an organism whose vulnerabilities contribute to shaping the specific clinical picture.

According to McKeown (1980), medical advances coincide with, rather than induce, the improvement of the health status of the population. His analysis of health and illness statistics of the late nineteenth century in England and Wales led him to conclude that the existence of healthier people and communities was not necessarily attributable to medical interventions but rather to factors such as improved nutrition, sounder environmental policies, and behavioral changes in the population. Visotsky et al. (1961) found that lifestyles could have a strong negative effect on health outcomes. Diet, tobacco use, alcohol consumption, irresponsible driving, noncompliance with prescribed medication intake, and responses to social pressures are some of the components of this equation. All of them are easily identifiable as culturally determined events.

Thus, alternative approaches to the strictly biomedical model point to socioeconomic and cultural factors as influencing physiological changes. The early observations of Cannon and Selye have been confirmed again and again by findings that environmental factors influence various parameters such as blood pressure and gastrointestinal, cardiovascular, and respiratory system functions, as well as neuroendocrine and immunological responses (Lipowski et al. 1977). Significant contributions in these areas are those by Hinkle (1973), as well as by others who concluded that disease episodes coincide with a threatening, disagreeable, demanding social environment.

Psychiatry's views about the pathogenesis of mental disorders have shifted over time, even though a traditional allegiance to the disease model was never substantially rejected (Akiskal and Webb 1978). Beyond psychoanalytic precepts, Levi and Kagan (1971) developed a theoretical model of disease as being produced by continuous feedback between various biological systems, mediated by well-identified psychosocial variables. Adamson and Schmale (1965) described the giving up/given up complex, a psychobiological process of "emotional defeat" that follows a loss in the interpersonal area. It has been demonstrated that excessive stress induces an enlargement of the adrenal glands and eventually the clinical phenomena of depression (Nemeroff et al. 1992). Many factors suggest the need to expand the scope of these studies: the impact of life events, the effect of social networks, and the phenomenology of widowhood, grief, bereavement, separations, environmental traumas, migration, uprootedness, and social disintegration. Ultimately, these factors also emphasize the interconnections between culture and medicine and culture and psychiatry (Kleinman 1988).

■ Brief Historical Review

The early work on what can be called classical cultural psychiatry appeared slightly over 100 years ago (Cooper 1934). Kraepelin (1904) is considered by many to be the precursor of transcultural or comparative psychiatry (Jilek 1995). The two main features of the early period were the focus on the "exotic"—unusual clinical syndromes seen in distant lands, most of them sites of colonial domination—and the universalistic interpretation of their findings. This initial research was seriously hampered by poor methodology, broad overgeneralizations, the absence of pilot studies, and interdisciplinary miscommunications, leading to unreliable conclusions.

The contributions of psychoanalysis were explicated by Freud in *Totem and Taboo* (Freud 1913/1955) and *Civilization and Its Discontents* (Freud 1922/1955). Dissidents like Jung and Adler and neo-Freudians such as Horney (1937) and Fromm (1978) considered sociocultural factors central to the genesis of human maladaptations and mental disorders (Zaphiropoulos 1982). During the 1940s and 1950s, American anthropologists and psychoanalysts, mainly based in New York's Columbia University, attempted a series of collaborative studies under the "Culture and Personality" theme; names such as Abraham Kardiner, Edward Sapir, Melford Spiro, and Weston La Barre conferred high respectability on this series of studies. Their work later evolved into the description of national characters via psychodynamic interpretations of ethnographic observations (Benedict 1935; Bock 1969; Opler 1959). These collaborative efforts ended when members of each discipline—including by then psychiatry, psychology, sociology, social work, and nursing—began following their own academic traditions and developed parallel, narrowly focused approaches in relative isolation.

A number of developments in the last 20–30 years have enlarged the field of cultural psychiatry, refining its purposes, tools, and accomplishments. The universal acceptance of Engel's (1980) biopsychosocial approach to the study of medical events strengthened the multifactorial views held by eclectic psychiatrists. Modern approaches profess a renewed emphasis on ethnographic research regarding cultural variables rather than assuming the universality of psychodynamic and sociological theories (Kleinman 1979; Littlewood 1990); these approaches recognize

the different contexts of the occurrence of clinical phenomena and discuss their advantages and limitations. The changing tenets of culture and
of the conceptual bases of clinical research contribute to understanding
nurture neither as a process of inevitable conditioning nor as a statement
of a mythical homogeneity among human groups. Similarly, psychiatrists
do not have to become anthropologists and anthropologists do not have
to be amateur psychiatrists. The doors to an enriching exchange between
these two disciplines have been opened, and there are reasons to believe
that real pathological phenomena will not be trivialized through a sense-
less "culturalization" nor that real cultural factors will be pathologized as
symptoms or syndromes (Alarcón and Ruiz 1995).

Modern psychiatry and other mental health disciplines are abandoning their traditional reluctance to accept and adopt cultural views in the
overall assessment of patients. The interweaving of biological predispositions and physiological sites with social phenomena and cultural contexts applies now not only to the elucidation and description of
symptoms but to diagnosis, pathogenesis, treatment, and the organization
of mental health services (Lewis-Fernandez and Kleinman 1995; Ruiz
1993). Culture permeates all clinical phenomena, every clinician-initiated
intervention, the nucleus of human experiences, and the response that
one's behavior evokes from others. With ideological battles put aside and
the patient becoming once again the central focus of clinical disciplines,
modern psychiatry embraces cultural knowledge as a pragmatic tool for
its multiple activities.

The work of many experts in this field has increased in recent decades. In 1969, the Board of Trustees of the American Psychiatric Association officially approved a position statement on the delineation of
transcultural psychiatry as a specialized field of study (American Psychiatric Association 1969). That document also outlined research possibili-
ties and clinical and social applications of findings from comparative
studies, epidemiological surveys, case reports, and treatment modalities
in various settings. Throughout the last three decades, growing areas of
study in transcultural psychiatry have included

- The interactions between culture and personality
- Conflict and problems in environments of rapid social change
- Attitudes and beliefs regarding behavioral deviance
- Communication styles
- Assessment of stress
- Cultural determinants of public policy

■ Recent Advances

Progress in the clinical applications of cultural psychiatry may be due not only to the pluralistic demographic growth of American society but also to the increased sophistication of students in these areas. As a result of this renewed interest, activity in the field of cultural psychiatry increased significantly during the 1980s and 1990s. In addition to those mentioned above, promising areas include

- Culture and the mind
- Clinical guidelines in cross-cultural mental health
- Applications of therapeutic techniques to various ethnic groups
- Ethnopsychopharmacology
- The cultural implications of the new managed care approaches in the delivery of care

(Draguns 1986; Fishman et al. 1993; Gaw 1995; Lefley 1990; Lu 1996; Pumariega et al. 1996). One of the most cogent developments is the impact of cultural principles on psychiatric diagnosis, now duly recognized in the two main psychiatric classification systems in the world, the American Psychiatric Association's (2000) Diagnostic and Statistical Manual of Mental Disorders, Text Revision (DSM-IV-TR), and the World Health Organization's (WHO's) tenth edition of the International Classification of Diseases (ICD-10) (World Health Organization 1993).

At the international level, a lack of interest in cultural factors during the 1980s, in spite of the emphasis on psychosocial strategies to achieve mental health goals delineated by WHO (Murphy 1982), has transformed into concentrated collaborative work. The United Nations declared 1996–2006 the Decade of Mental Health ("Mental illness" 1996). WHO is slowly but consistently overcoming the constraints of its political, intergovernmental nature. Thus, in collaboration with the World Bank, WHO has been using novel approaches to the estimation of the costs of mental illness in developing countries in order to mobilize governments in a more concrete way (Desjarlais et al. 1995). It is now generally accepted that all kinds of health problems have powerful social roots and consequences and that the elaboration of international mental health policies appears to be imperative. The recently published Surgeon General's report on mental health (U.S. Department of Health and Human Services 1999) and related documents recognize such principles as well as the American context.

In the educational arena, the main professional organizations in mental health—including the American Psychiatric Association (1997), the American Psychological Association (1993), the American Nursing Association (1996), and the Council of Social Work Education (1994)—have come forward with specific recognition of the value of, relevance of, and need for assessing cultural factors in their members' everyday work and academic and training enterprises. The National Institute of Mental Health (1988) sponsored a conference on improving training in psychological services for ethnic minorities; following the conference, strategies for the optimal implementation of cultural and ethnic standards in training programs were developed. Specific guidelines for providers of psychological services to ethnic, linguistic, and culturally diverse populations included the need to

• Incorporate and enforce the standards of training relevant to cultural and ethnic issues
• Develop and evaluate model curricula
• Recruit and develop a culturally sophisticated faculty

The APA's Practice Guidelines for the Treatment of Psychiatric Disorders (American Psychiatric Association 2000) include specific mention of cultural elements. One of the specific areas in which cultural psychiatry concepts could have a significant impact is the growing field of cultural competence in care-planning activities. Cultural competence comprises a set of congruent behaviors, attitudes, and policies that come together in a system, agency, or among individuals, which enables them to work effectively in cross-cultural situations (Manoleas 1995). It entails a variety of levels, depending on its degree of sophistication and efficiency. Developing culturally competent services addresses not only real needs of the populations served but also a marketing strategy to promote the system to all segments of the community. This approach suggests identification of risk population pools, targeted populations, and goals; establishment of partnerships; the actual development of services; and the evaluation of the system's critical success factors. Appropriate services would result in equitable outcomes, with benefits to providers, clients and customers, the systems of care, minority communities, funding agencies, and the taxpayer (Fishman et al. 1993; Cross et al. 1989; Lu 1996).

■ Essential Definitions

Culture is defined as a set of meanings, behavioral norms, and values used by members of a particular society as they construct their unique view of the world. These values or reference points include areas such as social relationships, language, nonverbal expression of thoughts and emotions, religious beliefs, moral thought, technology, and financial philosophy. Furthermore, culture is not a static notion but one that changes as it is taught by one generation to the next (Leighton 1967; González et al. 1995).

The definition of culture has been compounded by two other concepts, race and ethnicity. *Race* is, above all, a concept by which human beings have been designated or grouped primarily on the basis of general physiognomy. Although the validity of this concept is highly questionable, its impact on the individual and on groups has been intense, perhaps, on the one hand, because of its seeming reference to physical, biological, and genetic underpinnings, and on the other, because of the conflicting and sometimes passionate responses it generates among different groups. *Ethnicity,* in turn, refers to the subjective sense of belonging to a group of people with a common origin and with shared social and cultural beliefs and practices. It entails the notion of identity, and as such it needs to be examined as a source of data regarding an individual's self-image and intrapsychic life.

Cultural psychiatry can be defined as the discipline that deals with the description, definition, assessment, and management of all psychiatric conditions as they reflect and are subjected to the patterning influence of cultural factors in a biopsychosocial context. Cultural psychiatry uses concepts and instruments from social and biological sciences to advance a full understanding of psychopathology and its treatment.

One of the most serious theoretical debates in cultural psychiatry concerns the distinction between *disease* and *illness* (Alarcón and Ruiz 1995; Cohen 1961; Kleinman 1988). Disease, in the biological tradition, represents all the manifestations of ill health that seem to be a response to physiological causes and that are translated into symptoms and signs typical of nosological descriptions found in medical textbooks. Hence, the semantic domain of the concept of disease is the inward environment of the human body. By contrast, illness belongs to the sociocultural realm, dominated by the symbolic nature of the disease and its symptoms and signs and primarily represented by the subjective, emotional, behavioral, interpretive, and communicative responses of the individual affected by the disease. Consequently, any theory of illness embodies a cultural tenet, and, according to Fabrega (1989, 1991), it is an attribute of the social system, or more specifically of the medical system, from a particular society. Yet the formal body of knowledge that sustains the concept should be distinguished from the informal or folk system for the understanding of illness. Ultimately, the relationship between disease and illness can be explained as "a transformation from disordered bodily organ systems (i.e., disease) to negatively valued changes in behavior and function (i.e., illness)" (Fabrega 1991, p. 102). While the biological perspective maintains deterministic and universalistic views, cultural psychiatry promotes an intense dialectic interaction between biology and the socioenvironmental domain.

A number of conceptual and methodological issues in cultural psychiatry are yet to be solved. Although its foundations are epidemiological, clinical, and ethnographic, its purpose goes beyond such boundaries as it attempts to find the meaning of the illness experience, explanatory models, family responses, and so on. In some ways, the ongoing evolution of cultural psychiatry responds to Devereux's (1961) dictum that science may be pure or noncultural for a while but that "as soon as this pure science became respectable and indigenous, it acquired specifically cultural connotations and can be rapidly transformed into a kind of 'magical' science" (p. 372). This happens because history goes through processes of deculturalization followed after a while by reculturalization, the creation of a new cultural environment that permeates its products. In this context, Devereux submitted that a very scientific discovery becomes, as times passes, an additional "myth" in the Western world.

■ Clinical Dimensions of Cultural Psychiatry

The modern emphasis on clinically applicable concepts rather than on theoretical digressions has resulted in a growing understanding of the relevance of the clinical aspects of cultural psychiatry as a whole. There is a cultural edge in every clinical event, intervention, or interaction between the treating agent and the identified patient. These concepts do not apply, then, only to ethnic minorities or distant societies outside the Western world. As culture permeates every activity of all human beings across the world, and as the interaction between different human groups becomes closer and more enmeshed, it is important to delineate the cultural dimensions of contemporary clinical psychiatry.

Cultural Psychiatry Model and Five Functions of Culture

The model developed as a frame of reference for this topic includes five groups or types of functions of culture that are related to clinical psychopathology (Alarcón et al. 1999):

1. An interpretive and explanatory tool of behaviors that may or may not constitute clinical entities
2. A pathogenic and pathoplastic agent
3. A diagnostic and nosological factor
4. A protective and therapeutic instrument
5. An element in the management and structuring of clinical services

Interpretive and Explanatory Tool

The *interpretive and explanatory* role of culture emphasizes, for the most part, the nonpathological nature of human behavior, providing pertinent information to assist the clinician in understanding or even explaining the observed behaviors. Through this process, clinicians become familiar with culturally determined conditions that can assist them in making sense of situations that otherwise may lead to quick, facile, conclusive, and often mistaken clinical labeling—a process that often has highly stigmatizing power (Kirmayer 1989). Similarly, knowledge of the existence of cultural factors encourages the study of explanatory models of illness as provided by the patients themselves. Examples of this role of culture are the correct assessment of psychotic-like behaviors in some cultural groups, the meaning of somatic symptoms or dissociative states (Prince and Tcheng-Laroche 1987), and an objective assessment of behaviors that otherwise can be called "personality disorders" (Alarcón and Foulks 1995).

Pathogenic and Pathoplastic Agent

Furthermore, there is no question that culture can operate as both a *pathogenic* and a *pathoplastic* agent: cultural events or situations may generate, or may contribute to the causation of, abnormal behaviors. This conclusion is based on the literature on the deleterious effects of some child-rearing practices, family-based experiences, and even societal influences (including the powerful impact of the media) on the shaping of personalities, coping and response mechanisms, and other behaviors, particularly among the most vulnerable population segments (Fabrega 1990; Guarnaccia et al. 1993). Even more eloquent are examples of clinical conditions determined by cultural events such as warfare, interethnic hatred, and alcohol and drug consumption (Vaillant 1983; Wolf and Mosnaim 1990). Culture is also a pathoplastic agent because it modulates the symptomatic expression of a given clinical entity. Examples of this phenomenon can be seen in

- The content of some delusional and hallucinatory states mirroring contemporary personages, events, or trends
- The meaning of anxiety manifestations such as panic states (Lewis-Fernandez 1993)
- The messages carried by idioms of distress—that is, by "symptoms" that convey individual or collective messages of protest, discomfort, apathy, or resignation (Kleinman 1979)

Diagnostic and Nosological Factor

Culture is a powerful diagnostic and nosological factor in psychiatry. As a result of the work of many in the field, major contributions have made instruments such as DSM-IV (and DSM-IV-TR) and ICD-10 more culturally relevant. A pivotal concept is that of preventing the commission of a category fallacy—that is, the attempt to pigeonhole clinical entities or behaviors inherent in some cultures, societies, or human groups into the categories, models, or diagnostic terms advocated by the dominant classificatory systems (Csordas 1990; Kleinman 1979). One critical way that was devised to reach this objective was the proposal of a cultural formulation to describe the identity of the patient, his or her explanation of symptoms, the nature and functioning of the psychosocial environment, the diagnostician-patient relationship, and the overall assessment of cultural factors for diagnosis and care (Alarcón 1995; Fabrega 1987). The cultural formulation was introduced in DSM-IV (Fishman et al. 1993; Mezzich 1995), and it should become an important clinical and research tool in the field.

Therapeutic and Protective Role

There are well-documented examples of the *therapeutic and protective role* of culture in relation to psychopathological behaviors. The main point here is that culture and culturally determined attitudes and behaviors can operate as a cushion that prevents the occurrence of psychopathology and/or the spread of its harmful consequences. Findings of numerous studies on the role of extended families and social networks in neutralizing the impact of the stigma of mental illness or the isolation of the mentally ill are well known (Tung 1984; World Health Organization 1973). The traditional healing approaches and the role of religious beliefs and practices have proved to be potent auxiliary, yet not always secondary, sources of healing and health recovery (Fabrega and Mezzich 1987; Lukoff et al. 1995).

The vast research on culture and psychotherapy and the emerging field of ethnopsychopharmacology (Lin et al. 1993; Turner and Cooley-Quille 1996) testify to the growing importance of culture, including ethnicity, in this particular area. For instance, although federal legislation has recently mandated the inclusion of ethnic minorities and women as participants in pharmaceutical trials, psychopharmacological research in the United States—particularly when conducted or sponsored by pharmaceutical companies—has historically focused predominantly on young adult white males. One review (Turner and Cooley-Quille 1996) of the drug outcome studies published from 1991 to 1994 in four psychiatric journals (*American Journal of Psychiatry, Archives of General Psychiatry, Journal of Clinical Psychopharmacology,* and *Psychopharmacology Bulletin*) reported that, although the gender of research subjects was mentioned in 90% of studies, it was analyzed in an average of only 41%, and race/ethnicity was almost ignored (reported in 18% of subjects, analyzed in 8%). The relatively small number of studies that have investigated ethnic/racial differences in basic or clinical neuropsychopharmacology have been complicated by the fact that the broadly classified ethnocultural groups usually targeted (e.g., Asians, Hispanics) are composed of multiple subgroups that may differ significantly in a variety of genetic and environmental characteristics (e.g., Japanese versus Chinese versus Filipino; Mexican versus Caribbean versus South American).

Genetically determined racial/ethnic differences in psychopharmacology can result both from differences in liver function and metabolism and from differences in clinical responses to specific psychotropics (Lin et al. 1993). The identification of the cytochrome P450 enzyme systems and the subsequent categorization of most hepatically metabolized psychotropics has begun to promote clinicians' awareness of ethnoculturally determined responses. Similarly, ethnocultural factors have been identified across the range of responses to psychotropics, from inadequate dosing to toxic interactive effects. Many other psychosocial factors such as diet and nutrition; consumption of cigarettes, caffeine, alcohol, herbs, and other psychoactive substances; sleep or activity/rest patterns; and differences associated with environmental or geographical effects have also been found to influence ethnocultural differences in psychotropic metabolism and/or response (Jacobsen 1994).

Element in the Management and Structuring of Clinical Services

Culture is a critical element in the structure of *management approaches and provision of services* to large communities. Such approaches and such provision of services are based on the understanding and delineation of several concepts: 1) cultural sensitivity (awareness of culturally based needs in a given population), 2) cultural relevance (implementation of measures that help to provide culturally sensitive services), and 3) cultural competence, the ultimate product of such approaches and services, bolstered by good outcomes research documenting the benefits of the services provided (Cross et al. 1989).

Current demographic trends and legal immigration from various regions of the world provide dramatic information about the United States population on the eve of the twenty-first century. By the year 2020, the majority of the United States population will be composed of individuals from the so-called ethnic minorities (U.S. Bureau of the Census 1994). It is clear that the health care needs of this diverse population will reflect cultural factors brought in by the immigrants as well as those resulting from an uneven acculturation process. Basic administrative arrangements, physical plant designs, and the composition of culturally competent teams with well-identified case managers (some of them coming from the same cultural group as the consumers) make this role of culture extremely important in the contemporary health care scene (González et al. 1995).

Economy and social mobility have always reflected a number of cultural practices and have had, in turn, a decisive effect on the cultural changes taking place throughout history. Depending on the degree of education, technological sophistication, and collective development of the American population, culture can evolve into a constructive component of such evolution or may be distorted by conflict, dissension, and polarization. The current social climates in all the regions of the world require concerted action by psychiatrists and other mental health workers to disseminate the pragmatic and universal messages of clinically relevant cultural psychiatry. Every patient (actual or potential) in any geographic area, country, or society carries a cultural legacy as an indivisible part of his or her being. In times of disease and its concomitant psychosocial difficulties, such cultural factors become as powerful as the biological determinants of pathology and therefore require informed awareness and action by those responsible for the patient's care. It is important to maintain a culturally aware professional community to conduct an ongoing assessment of cultural factors in all aspects of its work.

That same professional community will continue leading the fight for destigmatization. Stigma is a deleterious cultural by-product in the consideration of mental illness and mental disorders. Culturally minded psychiatrists see this phenomenon as a clarion call to join forces with other professionals and professional organizations to achieve parity in insurance coverage, fairness in employment opportunities for mentally ill individuals, equal access to treatment and social development opportunities, and an end to other subtle and not-so-subtle discriminatory practices. Such ideas are reflected in the cultural variables examined in the next chapter as they create a frame for a genuine cultural assessment of clinical cases.

■ References

Adamson JD, Schmale AH: Object loss, giving up and the onset of psychiatric disease. Psychosom Med 27:557–576, 1965

Akiskal HS, Webb WL (eds): Psychiatric Diagnosis: Exploration of Biological Predictors. New York, SP Medical & Scientific Books, 1978

Alarcón RD: Culture and psychiatric diagnosis: impact on DSM-IV and ICD-10. Psychiatr Clin North Am 18:449–466, 1995

Alarcón RD, Foulks EF: Personality disorders and culture: contemporary clinical views. Cult Divers Ment Health 1:3–17, 1995

Alarcón RD, Ruiz P: Theory and practice of cultural psychiatry in the U.S. and abroad, in Review of Psychiatry. Edited by Oldham JM, Riba MB. Washington, DC, American Psychiatric Press, 1995, pp 599–626

Alarcón RD, Westermeyer J, Foulks EF, et al: Clinical relevance of contemporary cultural psychiatry. J Nerv Ment Dis 187:465–471, 1999

American Nursing Association: Guidelines for consideration of cultural factors in nursing education. Washington, DC, American Nursing Association, 1996.

American Psychiatric Association: Position statement on the delineation of Transcultural Psychiatry as a specialized field of study. Am J Psychiatry 126: 453–455, 1969

American Psychiatric Association: Diagnostic and Statistical Manual of Mental Disorders, 4th Edition. Washington, DC, American Psychiatric Association, 1994

American Psychiatric Association: Curricula Projects on Minority and Underrepresented Groups. Washington, DC, American Psychiatric Association, 1997

American Psychiatric Association: American Psychiatric Association Practice Guidelines for the Treatment of Psychiatric Disorders (Compendium 2000). Washington, DC, American Psychiatric Association, 2000

American Psychiatric Association: Diagnostic and Statistical Manual of Mental Disorders, 4th Edition, Text Revision. Washington, DC, American Psychiatric Association, 2000

American Psychological Association: Guidelines for providers of psychological service to ethnic, linguistic, and culturally diverse populations. Am Psychol 48:45–48, 1993

Benedict R: The Chrysanthemum and the Sword: Patterns of Japanese Culture. New York, Houghton Mifflin, 1935

Bock PK: Modern Cultural Anthropology. New York, Knopf, 1969

Cohen H: The evolution of the concept of disease, in Concepts of Medicine. Edited by Lush B. New York, Pergamon, 1961

Cooper JE: Diagnosis and the diagnostic process, in Handbook of Psychiatry. Edited by Shepherd M, Zangwill OL. Cambridge, UK, Cambridge University Press, 1983

Cooper JM: Mental disease situations in certain cultures: a new field for research. Journal of Abnormal Social Psychology 29:10–17, 1934

Council on Social Work Education: Accreditation Standards. Washington, DC, 1994

Cross TL, Bazron BJ, Dennis KW, et al: Towards a Culturally Competent System of Care: A Monograph on Effective Services for Minority Children Who Are Severely Emotionally Disturbed, Volume I. Washington, DC, Georgetown University Child Development Center, Child and Adolescent Service System Program (CASSP) Technical Assistance Center, 1989

Csordas TJ: Embodiment as a paradigm for anthropology. Ethos 18:5–47, 1990

Desjarlais R, Eisenberg L, Good B, et al: World Mental Health: Problems and Priorities in Low-Income Countries. New York, Oxford University Press, 1995

Devereux G: Cultural thought models in primitive and modern psychiatric theories. Psychiatry 24:359–374, 1961

Draguns JG: Culture and psycho-pathology: what is known about the relationship? Australian Journal of Psychology 38:329–338, 1986

Engel GL: The clinical application of the biopsychosocial model. Am J Psychiatry 137:535–543, 1980

Fabrega H: Psychiatric diagnosis: a cultural perspective. J Nerv Ment Dis 175:383–394, 1987

Fabrega H: Cultural relativism and psychiatric illness. J Nerv Ment Dis 177:415–425, 1989

Fabrega H: The concept of somatization as a cultural and historical product of Western medicine. Psychosom Med 52:653–672, 1990

Fabrega H: The culture and history of psychiatric stigma in early modern and modern Western societies: a review of recent literature. Compr Psychiatry 32:97–119, 1991

Fabrega H, Mezzich JE: Religion and secularization in psychiatric practice: three examples. Psychiatry 50:31–49, 1987

Fishman BM, Bobo L, Kosub K, et al: Cultural issues in serving minority populations: emphasis on Mexican-Americans and African-Americans. Am J Med Sci 306:160–166, 1993

Freud S: The Standard Edition of the Complete Psychological Works of Sigmund Freud. Translated and edited by Strachey J. London, Hogarth Press, 1955

Fromm E: Well Being of Man and Society. New York, Seabury, 1978

Gaw A (ed): Culture, Ethnicity, and Mental Illness. Washington, DC, American Psychiatric Press, 1995

González CA, Griffith EEH, Ruiz P: Cross-cultural issues in psychiatric treatment, in Treatment of Psychiatric Disorders, 2nd Edition, Vol 1. Edited by Gabbard GO. Washington, DC, American Psychiatric Press, 1995, pp 56–85

Guarnaccia PJ, Canino G, Rubio-Stipec M, et al: The prevalence of ataque de nervios in the Puerto Rico disaster study: the role of culture in psychiatric epidemiology. J Nerv Ment Dis 181:159–167, 1993

Hinkle LE: The concept of "stress" in the biological and social sciences. Science, Medicine and Man 1:31–48, 1973

Horney K: The Neurotic Personality of Our Time. New York, Norton, 1937

Jacobsen FM: Psychopharmacology and women of color, in Women of Color and Mental Health. Edited by Comas-Diaz L, Greene B. New York, Guilford 1994, pp 319–338

Jilek WG: Emil Kraepelin and comparative sociocultural psychiatry. Eur Arch Psychiatry Clin Neurosci 245:231–238, 1995

Kirmayer LJ: Cultural variations in the response to psychiatric disorders and emotional distress. Soc Science Med 29:327–339, 1989

Kleinman A: Patients and Healers in the Context of Culture. Berkeley, CA, University of California Press, 1979

Kleinman A: Rethinking Psychiatry: From Cultural Category to Personal Experience. New York, Free Press, 1988

Kraepelin E: Vergleichende psychiatrie (comparative psychiatry). Zentralblatt Nervenheilken Psychiatrie 27:433–443, 1904

Lefley HP: Culture and chronic mental illness. Hosp Comm Psychiatry 41:277–286, 1990

Leighton A: Is social environment a cause of psychiatric disorder? in Psychiatric Epidemiology and Mental Health Planning. Edited by Monroe RR, Klee GD, Brody EB. Psychiatric Research Report No 22, National Institute of Mental Health, Washington, DC, 1967

Levi L, Kagan A: Adaptation of the psycho-social environment to man's abilities and needs, in Society, Stress and Disease (Vol I). Edited by Levi L. London, Oxford University Press, 1971, pp 399–404

Lewis-Fernandez R: The role of culture in the configuration of dissociative states, in Dissociation, Culture, Mind and Body. Edited by Spiegel D. Washington, DC, American Psychiatric Press, 1993

Lewis-Fernandez R, Kleinman A: Cultural psychiatry: theoretical, clinical and research issues. Psychiatr Clin North Am 18:433–448, 1995

Lin KM, Poland RE, Nakasaki G (eds): Psychopharmacology and Psychobiology of Ethnicity. Washington, DC, American Psychiatric Press, 1993

Lipowski ZJ, Lipsitt DR, Whybrow PC (eds): Psychosomatic Medicine: Current Trends and Clinical Applications. New York, Oxford University Press, 1977

Littlewood R: From categories to contexts: a decade of the "new cross-cultural psychiatry." Br J Psychiatry 156:308–327, 1990

Lu FG: Getting to cultural competence: Guidelines and resources. Behav Health Care Tomorrow 3: 39–52, 1996

Lukoff D, Lu FG, Turner R: Cultural consideration in the assessment and treatment of religious and spiritual problems. Psychiatr Clin North Am 18: 467–486, 1995

Manoleas P: The Cross-Cultural Practice of Clinical Case Management in Mental Health. New York, Haworth Press, 1995

McKeown T: The Role of Medicine. Princeton, NJ, Princeton University Press, 1980

Mental illness to be among most prevalent by 2020, WHO study says. Psychiatric Times 13:1, 1996

Mezzich JE: Cultural formulation and comprehensive diagnosis: clinical and research perspectives. Psychiatr Clin North Am 1995; 18:649–658

Murphy HBM: Comparative Psychiatry: The International and Intercultural Distribution of Mental Illness. New York, Springer, 1982

National Institute of Mental Health: Proceedings of the Conference on Improving Training and Psychological Services for Ethnic Minorities, Washington, DC, October 1988. Rockville, MD, National Institute of Mental Health, 1988

Nemeroff CB, Krishnan KKR, Reed D, et al: Adrenal gland enlargement in major depression: a computed tomographic study. Arch Gen Psychiatry 49:384–387, 1992

Opler MK (ed): Culture and Mental Health. New York, MacMillan, 1959

Prince R, Tcheng-Laroche F: Culture-bound syndromes and international disease classification. Culture, Medicine and Psychiatry 11:3–11, 1987

Pumariega AJ, Diamond J, England MJ, et al: Best Principles for Managed Medicaid RFPs. Washington, DC, American Academy of Child and Adolescent Psychiatry (Task Force on Community-Based Systems of Care), 1996

Ruiz P: Access to health care for uninsured Hispanics: policy recommendations. Hosp Comm Psychiatry 44:958–962, 1993

Tung M: Life values, psychotherapy, and East-West integration. Psychiatry 47:285–292, 1984

Turner SM, Cooley-Quille MR: Socioecological and sociocultural variables in psychopharmacological research: methodological considerations. Psychopharmacol Bull 32:183–192, 1996

U.S. Bureau of the Census: Current Population Reports, Series P-20. Washington, DC, U.S. Bureau of the Census, 1994

U.S. Department of Health and Human Services: Mental Health: A Report of the Surgeon General—Executive Summary. Rockville, MD, U.S. Department of Health and Human Services, Substance Abuse and Mental Health Services Administration, Center for Mental Health Services, National Institutes of Health, National Institute of Mental Health, 1999

Vaillant GE: The Natural History of Alcoholism. Cambridge, MA, Harvard University Press, 1983

Visotsky HM, Hamburg DA, Goss ME, et al: Coping behavior under extreme stress. Arch Gen Psychiatry 5:423–443, 1961

Wolf ME, Mosnaim AD (eds): Posttraumatic Stress Disorder: Etiology, Phenomenology and Treatment. Washington, DC, American Psychiatric Press, 1990

World Health Organization: The International Pilot Study of Schizophrenia. Geneva, World Health Organization, 1973

World Health Organization: International Classification of Diseases, 10th Edition. Geneva, World Health Organization, 1993

Zaphiropoulos ML: Transcultural parameters in the transference and countertransference. J Am Acad Psychoanal 10:571–584, 1982

2

Cultural Variables

Cultural factors interact with and are molded by the specific historical experiences of the patient as well as by his or her race, gender, age, values and belief systems, country of origin, family migration events, language, and social and ethnic factors, with their resulting degrees of discrimination and disenfranchisement. Throughout the patient's life, these variables interact to shape what ultimately becomes a personal identity. This chapter explores the nature, content, and effect of the most relevant cultural variables.

A patient's history can be approached in terms of his or her personal, family, and cultural evolvement. This history is possessed by the patient as constructs that can be detected by the use of key words uttered over and over as he or she interacts with the clinician. Kelly (1955) noted that cultural background can be elicited from the patient's personal explanation and the assigned meaning of the family's developmental history through generations. Another method of eliciting cultural identity is by using an interpersonal matrix, which involves assessing the patient's viewpoint about particular areas—such as demographics (age, gender, and location), status (social, educational, and economic), and affiliations (ethnic, religious, and family)—and the behaviors, expectations, and values associated with these factors (Pedersen and Ivey 1993). This model helps the clinician understand that behavior can have different meanings, depending on the patient's ethnic identity and cultural perspective (Westermeyer 1993).

■ Ethnic Identity

From the time of birth, and perhaps even before, the identity of the child is shaped and molded by a particular cultural milieu. Both language and culture are learned from early childhood and are elaborated and refined in adulthood. The recurrent patterns of an individual's preoccupations, memories, value judgments, attitudes, ambitions, and emotional responses are all facets of identity that are influenced by past and present cultural environments. One's thoughts and behavior are continually being overtly and covertly shaped by culture. Culture is omnipresent and, like language, is sometimes conscious and intentional (as seen in formal didactic education) and sometimes subtle and implicit in particular social surroundings. Culture also gives meaning to suffering in times of distress and provides the metaphors that lead to unique expressions of such suffering. In some cultures, stresses within the family may be ignored or unacknowledged because of shame or threat of disrupting traditional values. In these cases, symptoms may be instead manifested somatically or be attributed to spiritual forces or fate. Cultural patterns may promote behavioral responses such as drinking alcohol and thereby avoiding the stresses of family life.

The Cultural Formulation appended to DSM-IV-TR (American Psychiatric Association 2000, Appendix I) recommends that the clinician assess the ethnic identity of the patient as the first step in the process of diagnosis. This recommendation might seem familiar to most physicians, as they have traditionally been taught to do patient work-ups by starting with "Identifying Information and Chief Complaint." Most clinical presentations begin with the phrase, "the patient is a 42-year-old black male who…" or "is a 12-year-old white female who…" or "is a 73-year-old Hispanic male who…" Such descriptors are taken for granted and by now have become almost universal in clinical conferences, ward rounds, and case reports.

Eliciting the patient's self-perception of his or her own ethnic identity is an important procedure in the diagnostic process and is also helpful in designing the treatment and management interactions that follow. How then does the physician validly describe the ethnic identity of the patient? The first step in this process is to ask the patient about cultural and religious backgrounds. Notice that the plural "backgrounds" is used, for the patient's mother and father may have different cultural origins. People who live in multicultural societies may have several ethnic traditions from which much of their identity is derived. In patients from minority cultural backgrounds, the identity acquired by the process of enculturating to mainstream American culture adds another layer of complexity, the one derived from the family's moving from place to place. Growing up in different neighborhoods and in different countries can add complex dimensions to ethnic identification. The dynamics of cultural influences in forming identity are as complex as are psychodynamics in the formation of personality. Although patients may be able to articulate some cultural influences with full awareness, others may be so automatic and taken for granted that they are discoverable only by studied self-reflection and inference. In nearly all such cases, terms we commonly use to categorize ethnicity may be simplistic.

Giving the patient the opportunity to reflect on personal cultural identification may allow for expressions that affirm the self and inform the clinician. Several caveats, however, must be considered in the process of assigning ethnic identity labels to a patient. Much of the terminology now in official and common use to designate ethnic identity is actually quite questionable from a scientific perspective. For example, the ethnic categorizations of people as black, Hispanic, Asian, and American Indian lack comparability with one another because each category has different referents. *Black* refers to a color, *Hispanic* to a language, *Asian* to a continent, and *American Indian* to a heterogeneous group of aboriginal peoples in the United States.

Distinctions based on skin color have been used for purposes of social discrimination, oppression, and segregation. During Reconstruction after the Civil War, many families in the southern states were divided arbitrarily, using the criterion of shade of skin color. Family members who could pass as white were considered white, and those of darker hue were called colored, Negro, or black. This issue remains problematic to their descendants to this day. Skin color is in fact a poor marker of ethnic or genetic differentiation. Physical anthropologists in Nazi Germany lumped people of dark brown complexion in Africa, South India, Melanesia, and Australia into the same general racial group, termed Negroid. These different populations were erroneously believed to be somehow genetically connected in prehistory. The international Human Genome Project has recently demonstrated that African populations are, in fact, closer to European in genetic configuration. Melanesians and Aborigines share more genetic patterns with Southeast Asians than with Africans of similar skin tone!

Hispanic is another ethnic designator that, although used as a political banner for many disenfranchised Americans, has (like skin color) dubious validity in determining ethnicity. Hispanics, Hispanic Americans, and Latinos tend to be labeled as such regardless of country of origin and cultural background, thereby leading to clinical and research categories that are virtually meaningless. A variety of cultural variables such as language, race, ethnicity, religious and spiritual beliefs, dietary habits, folk beliefs and tradition, cultural identity, and social outlooks vary greatly among the many Hispanic ethnic subgroups who reside in the United States. *Hispanic* presumably can apply to people from both Spain and South America who speak Spanish. Are Spanish-speaking Filipinos to be considered Hispanic or Asian? Are Brazilians who speak Portuguese also Hispanics? Consider the cultural and possible genetic variability between Argentinians of European Jewish descent, Puerto Ricans of Afro-Caribbean descent, and Mexicans of Mayan Indian descent. Yet all speak Spanish and are from Latin America. From the perspective of a racial grouping based on skin color, one group could be considered white, another black, and the third red.

Designations based on geographical place of origin are also inadequate indicators of ethnic identity. *Caucasian, American Indian, Asian American,* and *African American* are examples of general categories used for this purpose. *Caucasian* presumably refers to white people of European ancestry, but the term would probably exclude populations with epicanthic folds who actually live in the region of the Caucasus mountains of Central Asia. *American Indian,* on the other hand, refers to people from 260 different language groups, some descended from groups that migrated from North Asia during the last Ice Age. Other populations considered to be in this category, such as the Inuit (Eskimos), migrated more recently—between 5,000 years ago and the present (witness recent migrations of Eskimos from Siberia to Alaska). These rather recent arrivals from Asian Siberia are not, however, considered Asian Americans.

The term *Asian American* commonly refers to people coming from Far Eastern countries such as Japan, China, Korea, and countries of Southeast Asia (Vietnam, Cambodia, Laos, Thailand). Asians from India, Pakistan, Iran, Iraq, Turkey, and other Near Eastern or Middle Eastern countries are usually not included in this category. Although numerous people in the United States are often referred to as Muslims (a religious preference) or Middle Easterners, they have not as yet been categorized as an official ethnic minority. It is obvious that these various populations in Asia are as diverse ethnically, religiously, and linguistically as are Native Americans. For example, the spiritualist Hmong, Catholic Vietnamese, and Buddhist Chinese, all living in Vietnam, are divergent in religion, language, racial attributions, and history.

If the clinician does not actively explore these issues during the interviewing process, attributing racial and ethnic identities to the patient may be invalid and may even have pernicious results. For example, arbitrarily classifying patients according to perceived skin tone may not only identify but also reinforce historically derived categories of social discrimination and negative stereotyping. Therefore, clinicians need to be aware of and actively inquire about the patients' self-attributions regarding ethnicity, race, social class, and religion. By exploring each of these items, the clinician can develop mutual understandings with the patient in regard to cultural and social influences on the patient's mental disorder and its treatment.

■ Race

As implied above, there is no ready consensus today on what is meant by *race*. When considered as a biological phenomenon, it is obvious, for example, that there is relatively little agreement on what is actually meant by *black* or *white*. The genetic heterogeneity of American society makes it impossible to define lucidly what is meant by any race-linked terminology. Furthermore, census law, years ago in the southern United States, establishing that a drop of "black blood" made an individual black, was specious hopefulness. Stories were well known, for example, of one light-skinned woman's living as a black in one community while the woman's equally light-skinned sibling was living as a white in a community where no one had knowledge of the family's relations. Therefore such preoccupations were not with the genetic concept but with the phenotypic expression, particularly as translated into skin color.

Despite this lack of precision and clarity with respect to racial classifications, race has assumed particular significance in the United States: the historical American experience with slavery has led to the clear linkage of stereotyped concepts and stigmata to black skin. On the other hand, notions of superiority and intellectual cleverness have come to be associated with white skin. In a similar fashion, characteristics that are more or less valued by American society have been linked to individuals classified as bearing the external markers of the Mongoloid groups (for example, the Native Americans and the Chinese).

The complexity of grouping people together on the basis of race is compounded by individuals' willingness to come together because they share a common cultural heritage. Hence, blacks can indeed look very different but still agree that they are African American in cultural outlook. Furthermore, it is only relatively recently that the notion of substantive variability in ethnic identity among blacks has taken on currency: thus one dark-skinned individual may be minimally Afrocentric and may be conservative in political outlook, whereas another equally dark-skinned person may be resolutely Afrocentric and a political liberal. Cross (1991) has also argued that an individual may change ethnic identity over his or her adult life.

In American society, many individuals are faced with the tasks of ultimately consolidating a racial and an ethnic identity. Regarding racial identity, it is not enough to decide whether one is black or white. It is also of some import whether one agrees, for example, with the concept that *black* should be equated with a model of deficiency and inferiority. The task of formulating an ethnic identity has considerably broader implications because it relates to establishing identification with a large number of values important in society.

Race as a powerful factor in American life is practically ubiquitous in its effects, and the potentially problematic interaction between different racial groups is a significant element in practically every facet of life. Not surprisingly, therefore, clinicians have come to recognize that race has some importance in the context of psychiatric practice. Bradshaw (1982) argued cogently that the patient–clinician dyad and the clinician–supervisor dyad were substantively influenced by racial considerations. Race can affect clinical understanding, with significant consequences for the diagnostic process and ultimately for treatment decisions.

More than one author (Adebimpe 1981; Jones and Gray 1986) has pointed out how psychiatric disorders in blacks are frequently misdiagnosed. Blacks are more frequently diagnosed with schizophrenia, and less often diagnosed with mood disorders, than are whites. It is assumed that these diagnostic differences are based on cultural differences in language and interaction styles, values, and methods of communication between patient and clinician.

Flaskerud and Hu (1992) studied a sample of more than 26,000 patients of the Los Angeles County mental health system and found that whites and Asians more often received the diagnoses of major affective disorders than did blacks or Hispanics and that blacks and Asians received the diagnoses of schizophrenia and other psychoses more often than did whites. The authors concluded that differential diagnosis decisions in psychiatry may be related to factors of race and ethnicity. The question of why blacks continue to receive a diagnosis of depression less frequently than do whites remains unanswered. It may be that depression in blacks is manifested with more anger than in other groups, or that it is more difficult for some clinicians to establish the kind of relationship with black patients that allows the clinician to understand black patients' depressive features. Furthermore, Newhill (1990) pointed out that the symptom of paranoia is not always indicative of psychopathology. Rather, it could sometimes be an adaptive mechanism employed by minority groups afflicted by low socioeconomic status, poor education, racial discrimination, and other sociocultural ills. Newhill recalled the notion of "healthy cultural paranoia," developed earlier by Grier and Cobbs (1968) and pointed out that the thoughtful clinician must learn to distinguish cautious suspiciousness that is functionally adaptive from paranoid illness. There are also diagnostic dilemmas posed by bereaved Hispanic or Native American patients who describe the experience of hearing a deceased relative's voice. The auditory hallucination in this context is not always a symptom of psychotic depression but may simply be a culturally sanctioned expression of uncomplicated bereavement.

Last and Perrin (1993) conducted a comparative study of black and white children brought for treatment of an anxiety disorder. The results suggested that, although the two groups of children were more clinically similar than different, the black children were more likely to suffer from posttraumatic stress disorder. Urban populations of black children may be exposed to more violence than may whites. Fabrega et al. (1993) studied a cohort of black and white adolescents at a public university-based clinic. They found that eating disorders were more common among whites, whereas conduct disorders were more common among blacks. The authors considered the possibility that referral bias could have explained some of their findings. Eating disorders may be in some way more bound to certain cultures (Brumberg 1989). It has also been observed, however, that nonblack clinicians are more prone to diagnose conduct disorder in black youth and antisocial personality disorder in black adult males (Brumberg 1989).

It is useful for clinicians to understand that those called blacks in the United States are culturally heterogeneous, with traditions originating in various parts of the world, such as Africa and the Caribbean. Because of this varied cultural influence, many individuals may embody, as Kirmayer (1989) termed it, "a cultural variation in the response to emotional distress." Littlewood (1985) has described an example of such variations in the syndrome among Trinidadian men called *tabanka*, observed in a man who has been deserted by his wife for another man. He responds by wandering aimlessly about or remaining alone at home, feeling worthless, harboring angry feelings about the wife, and complaining of insomnia and anhedonia. Littlewood viewed this syndrome as a manifestation of depression. However, its strangeness in the American context could easily lead an unsuspecting clinician to view it as a psychotic disorder.

Comas-Diaz and Jacobsen (1991) thoughtfully delineated the influence of race and ethnicity on the therapeutic context. For example, they pointed out the tendency toward projective identification, a so-called primitive defense mechanism, wherein the patient attributes to the therapist certain qualities that are characteristic of the patient's own racial and cultural identity. Such natural transferential distortion in the therapy process may also be encountered in diagnosis. Race is an important element in clinical psychiatric practice that may have an effect on the process of engaging the patient, assessment of psychopathology, and creation and implementation of the treatment plan.

■ Gender and Sexual Orientation

Like race, gender is a core factor in the formation of cultural identity. From the moment of authoritative labeling of an infant as girl or boy, society categorizes the individual and dictates expectations and behaviors as masculine or feminine. This influences how boys and girls are related to by their parents and the society at large and thus shapes their sense of themselves and their modes of functioning and relating to others, including the examining physician. The formation of gender identity is a developmental achievement, multidetermined by biological, psychological, and sociocultural factors, that results in the self-representation, awareness, and cognitive understanding of oneself as man or woman (Moore and Fine 1990).

Gender roles and behaviors as a cultural variable are not in and of themselves pathological. Nevertheless, from generation to generation, sociocultural influences have a significant impact on the development, cognitive identification, learned behaviors, role functioning, and social expectations of males and females, based on their identified gender. Stein (1993) extensively reviewed the development and meaning of lesbian, gay, and bisexual identities, which add to these individuals' gender issues those of yet another minority group in society. Stein also outlined assessment and treatment implications for persons with these sexual orientations across ethnic, age, and class groups to acknowledge the synergistic effect of these aspects of cultural identity.

DSM-IV (and its text revision DSM-IV-TR) discusses gender as a variable in the prevalence and the clinical presentation of disorders preceding the consideration of diagnosis. Certain disorders generally tend to be more common in one gender than in the other. For example, mental retardation, reading and language disorders, autistic disorders, attention-deficit/hyperactivity disorder (ADHD) and conduct disorders (before puberty) are more common in boys; alcohol abuse and dependence, most substance-related disorders (except cocaine), gender identity disorders, impulse control disorders, obsessive-compulsive disorder (OCD), and specific personality disorders (e.g., antisocial) are more common in men. The paraphilias occur almost exclusively in males and are extremely rare in females. On the other hand, mood and anxiety disorders, conversion disorders, dissociative disorders, pain disorders, and other personality disorders—such as borderline, histrionic, and dependent—are more frequently diagnosed in women. Anorexia and bulimia nervosa occur almost exclusively in women and are rare in males. Other disorders occur equally in both males and females. These include feeding disorders of infancy and early childhood, separation anxiety disorders, bipolar disorders, dysthymic disorder, adjustment disorders, hypochondriasis, cocaine abuse, and certain personality disorders—for example, the avoidant type.

Although gender as a cultural variable may determine the epidemiological prevalence of certain diagnostic categories, there are also differences in prevalence in clinical samples. This may be the result of gender differences in acknowledgment or denial of symptoms, in differential treatment-seeking behaviors, or in biases in diagnosing. Additionally, ethnicity is a factor in gender variations. For example, whereas Latino men have somewhat higher rates of alcohol abuse and dependence than do white and African American men, Latino women have lower rates of these disorders than do women from any other ethnic group.

DSM-IV-TR suggests other possible confounding issues regarding gender. For example, although clinical studies suggest higher incidences of separation anxiety disorders, social phobias, and generalized anxiety disorders in women, these statistics are not borne out by epidemiological surveys, which may suggest differences in treatment-seeking behaviors and/or denial of certain symptoms in men. Similarly, it is unclear whether differences in the prevalence of diagnosis of certain personality disorders (e.g., antisocial in men and histrionic in women) represent real gender differences or expected, stereotypical behaviors (aggression in men and seductiveness in women). When making a psychiatric diagnosis it is important to consider gender and its stereotypes regarding socially appropriate roles and behavior.

Gender is also a cultural variable that may influence onset, clinical presentation, course, and treatment-seeking behavior. For example, Fullilove (1993) discussed how minority women's status affects health, sexual practices, and the locus of treatment. In addition, Comas-Diaz and Greene (1994) stressed the heterogeneity of these issues in different groups of women and integrated culturally relevant and gender-sensitive issues into guidelines for clinical practice with African American, Latina or Hispanic, Asian American, American Indian, West Indian, and East Indian women.

Although the clinician must be cautious about stereotyping, it is, on the other hand, important to be aware of issues that are dynamically significant in the psychology of men and women and of how these issues influence their concepts of self and their relationships with others. These factors have important implications for understanding the nature of the therapeutic relationship that develops (often based on the gender of patient and of therapist), as well as the nature of the issues that may be most psychologically relevant in the life of the patient because of his or her gender.

There is considerable evidence from history, art, and literature in Western countries that the greatest struggle for men is protecting themselves from anything that would diminish masculine pride (e.g., manliness, *machismo, menschlichkeit,* manly courage, balls, *huevos*). In fact, the ideal of masculinity in most cultures is a man who is assertive, active, independent, self-reliant, and unemotional (Notman and Nadelson 1991). Masculine pride is often maintained through continual quests for money, power, recognition, and status. Astrachan (1988) clearly illustrates these features in his examination of the dynamic struggles of men challenged with coping and adapting to women's emerging quest for independence, equality, and power over the past few decades. Such values may lead patients to deny or minimize symptoms or need more time feeling secure enough to acknowledge deep-seated anxieties and fears. Fears of being unmanly and desire for the rewards of achieving standards of masculinity have always been more important issues in the psychology and lives of men than their counterpart issues have been for women (Stoller 1968).

For many men, relying on others to help them solve their problems may generate conflicts about helplessness and dependency, making them feel weakened or "less than a man." Passivity, fear of merger, and fear of reengulfment are issues that most men continue to struggle with as a remnant of early rapprochement struggles to ward off the dangerous "mother after separation" (Mahler et al. 1975). How these issues manifest themselves with a female therapist and with a male therapist may be quite different. Discussion of these topics, however, become a central resistance in treatment and have to be worked through to facilitate the male patient's settling into therapy, acknowledging important issues and associated affects, and making good use of the therapist and of the therapeutic relationship.

Despite individual endowments, capacities, or achievements, women in Western countries have been observed to be more motivated by emotional connectedness and relationships than are men (Comas-Diaz and Greene 1994). As Clower (1991) and others have suggested, the vicissitudes in the psychological development of females lead to some very positive capabilities—for example, flexibility in adaptive regression, identification, empathy, affiliation, and close intimacy. On the other hand, females may have liabilities: low self-esteem, inhibition of independence and self-assertion, and a proclivity to endure less than satisfying relationships (with males and/or females). Mass media and other areas of society also offer contradictory messages to females that encumber their attempts to sustain self-esteem (Bland 1994).

Female reactions to real or perceived separation or loss may be more central and intense than those experienced by males. Women may be more sensitive to the experience of loss at developmental points that are crucial in the movement toward autonomy and independence (e.g., leaving home, graduation, new job), as well as at the point of initiating or terminating a relationship. In the treatment relationship, this female propensity for connectedness (which serves them in their maternal roles) may tend to become so invested in the therapeutic relationship that it undermines their ability to be forthcoming and to reveal their true self. Females may be more prone to seek approval and acceptance, downplaying their strengths and resourcefulness. Underlying their complaints of depression and anxiety (often a generic idiom) may be the return of unresolved issues around separation-individuation. This problem, when influenced by current events in their lives, can result in women's becoming demoralized and in having difficulty regulating self-esteem. When the clinician too readily colludes with this sense of helplessness, it may inhibit the progressive working through of unresolved issues, maturation, and the consolidation of the sense of self and of personal competency.

■ Age

As is the case with gender, age interacts with the other components of cultural identity to influence developmental issues, as well as the psychiatric assessment and treatment of any individual patient. For example, Canino and Spurlock (1994) discussed working with economically disadvantaged children and adolescents from culturally diverse backgrounds, recognizing the significance of cultural variations in help-seeking behavior, discrimination, and socioeconomic pressures on adaptive responses and mental health. They found that children and adolescents from ethnic minorities may show variations in symptoms of mental illness resulting from family structure, family interaction, and role identification. Similarly, older ethnic minority patients may also show variations in presentation of symptoms. Yamamoto (1982) has described Japanese being socialized to behave in a respectful, proper, and deferential manner, which often results in inhibition about revealing symptoms of depression to an authority figure such as a psychiatrist.

The American Psychiatric Association (1994) Task Force on Ethnic Minority Elderly has presented specific outlines for clinical care of the elderly from the four major ethnic minority groups. In all groups, elderly persons feel the losses of migration more keenly than do other age groups because they leave behind more years of memories and connections than do the younger immigrants. Migration at a later stage of life is handicapped by a lesser ability to acculturate and a higher risk of culture shock (Sakauye 1992). Elderly persons are more likely to manifest "culture-bound syndromes," which creates difficulties in diagnosis. Also confounding the diagnostic process is the fact that many speak only their native languages. Ethnic-minority elderly persons may also feel displaced in Western societies, in which aged persons may be abandoned or placed in nursing homes.

Other issues encountered in the psychiatric context with ethnic-minority elderly groups (Lukoff et al. 1992; Sakauye 1992) include

- The overdiagnosis of schizophrenia and dementia in African Americans
- The poor use of services by Asian persons as a result of poor education, superstition, and fear of Western medications
- Similar underuse by Hispanic individuals as a result of feared social stigma
- In Native Americans, the tendency to rely on traditional healers whose beliefs are poorly understood by Western clinicians

■ Religion

Religious and spiritual beliefs profoundly influence mental status as well as psychiatric assessment and treatment (Larson 1993; Lukoff et al. 1992, 1992a, 1993). Included in DSM-IV-TR's nonillness category ("Additional Conditions That May Be a Focus of Clinical Attention") is "Religious or Spiritual Problem" (p. 741). It is important for the clinician to acknowledge and work with religious beliefs as potential sources of support rather than only as manifestations of psychopathology. For example, Browning et al. (1990) write about the therapeutic effects of the Protestant, Jewish, and Roman Catholic religious perspectives. Griffith and Young (1988) also describe therapeutic aspects of Christian religious rituals in African Americans. In addition, Burton (1992) examined the interactions between religion and family as resources that could be assessed and used.

From another perspective, religious explanations of mental illnesses often involve supernatural or spiritual causation. For example, Mexican Americans as well as the Navajo people of Arizona and New Mexico attribute the origin of disease to spells, often referred to as *embrujo* (bewitchment), caused by witches (Kluckhohn 1967; Madsen 1973). In these cultural groups, a person who experiences a stressful event such as disease or the accidental death of a child may attribute the experience to the magical powers of a witch who has put a hex on the victim. The Raramuri Indians of northern Mexico believe that multiple soul entities that are responsible for human behavior inhabit every person's body. According to the Raramuri, there are *large souls* that control important mental functions such as cognition, whereas less complicated *smaller souls* control bodily functions such as movement of the limbs. This theory of behavior also explains abnormal states such as drunkenness. The Raramuri believe that alcohol causes the large, mature souls to depart from the body, leaving only small, undisciplined souls and resulting in the irrational behaviors commonly associated with alcohol intoxication. They believe that if the large souls do not return to the body, the affected individual will experience a chronic irrational state such as psychosis. Furthermore, a person may become physically ill and even die if the large souls do not return (Merrill 1988).

Kleinman (1988) has termed such theories "explanatory models of illness." The explanatory model may consist of unique notions of etiology, timing, mode of onset, pathophysiology, natural history, severity, and appropriate treatments. Psychological causation is an example of the explanatory model in the Western patient, whereas a broken taboo may be the explanation used by some traditional Native Americans. The Native American patient may also experience hearing the voice of a dead person calling to him or her as the spirit travels to the afterworld. If the clinician were unaware of such a spiritual belief, the patient might be thought to have psychotic symptoms. Clinicians can elicit the explanatory model by asking the patient "What has happened?" "Why?" and "Why now?" The clinician should also ask "What will happen if nothing is done?" and "What effect will the experience have on others?" Finally, the clinician should ask "What can be done about it?" in order to lay the foundation of a therapeutic plan that includes pertinent cultural considerations.

Cultural explanations also affect help-seeking behavior. The preferred diagnostic and treatment strategies may be partially fashioned according to the patient's explanatory model of illness (Kleinman 1988; McGoldrick et al. 1982; Rogler and Cortés 1993). For example, because some patients intentionally act healthier than they actually are in order to avoid the cultural stigma of their illness, it is sometimes necessary to speak with a collateral informant to obtain an accurate history. Family and other informants, of course, may also minimize symptoms because of the stigma involved in seeking assistance for mental disorders.

Among some Asian groups, such as Chinese and Japanese, a healthy and balanced life may depend on respect for family elders and the practice of ancestor worship (Gaw 1993). A typical response from a traditional Chinese family attempting to find help for a mental problem might include consultation with trusted elders and friends. The family might then seek herbalists and acupuncturists or consult a religious person. In most cases, they would present the illness in terms of somatic complaints. Other indigenous healing practitioners may also be used—such as *curanderos,* shamans, medicine men, and fortune-tellers (Gaines 1991). Often, the last resort when all else fails is turning to the Western clinic or hospital for help (Lin and Lin 1981).

■ Migration and Country of Origin

The psychosocial history of a recent immigrant should include the story of his or her exodus (Lee 1990). Salient factors of this story include country of origin, position in the family, education, employment status, level of support, political issues, experiences of war, and traumatic events. The clinician's goal is to understand a patient's baseline life experience in the country of origin. The history should also include details regarding the reasons for leaving, who was left behind, who paid for the trip, and any hardships and trauma suffered, including experiences of deprivation, torture, beatings, starvation, rape, or imprisonment. Migrants leave their countries voluntarily, and often easily, whereas refugees are either forced out or flee the country surreptitiously and may experience trauma and losses. Clinicians should also discuss the extent of the patient's

- Loss of family members, relatives, and friends
- Loss of property, financial resources, business, and career
- Loss of support of the cultural milieu, community, and religion

Immigration and country of origin can also influence mental health positively in certain populations. For example, Karno et al. (1987) compared Mexicans of American birth and Mexican birth using the Diagnostic Interview Schedule, Version III (DIS-III). They found that Mexican immigrants to California had fewer psychiatric conditions than did respondents of Mexican descent born in America. The United States–born Mexican Americans actually had a higher prevalence of psychiatric disorders, including abuse of alcohol and drugs, than did the general population in Los Angeles. Other research found that Chinese Americans experience depression at a lower prevalence than that found in Americans in general responding to epidemiological surveys (Sue et al. 1992; D. Takeuchi, S. Sue, and K. Kurasaki, "Chinese American Psychiatric Epidemiological Survey (CAPES)," unpublished document, 1994).

■ Socioeconomic Status

Poverty limits opportunities and expectations and contributes to psychopathology. Many ethnic groups that have migrated to the United States (U.S. Bureau of the Census 1993) have not fared as well economically as the majority culture, as reflected in the figures of the last two official censuses in the country (1990 and 2000). (See Tables 1 and 2.)

Fried (1982) reported that socioeconomically disadvantaged people experience a reduction in effective means of coping, which leads to a sense of helplessness and powerlessness. This reduction in coping skills may be related to the findings of psychopathology rates about two and one-half times the rates found in the highest socioeconomic groups (Dohrenwend et al. 1980).

Langner et al. (1974) found that while children of families on welfare were more severely impaired in health status than nonwelfare children,

TABLE 1. Economic status of different groups of ethnic minority immigrants in the United States

Ethnic group	Economic level (%)		
	Lower blue-collar	Poverty rate	Public assistance
Haitians	21.0	21.0	9.3
Jamaicans	11.0	12.1	7.8
Mexicans	32.0	29.7	11.3
Mexican Americans	19.0	24.5	13.5
Puerto Ricans	21.0	31.7	26.9
Nicaraguans	24.0	24.4	8.4
Salvadorans	27.0	24.9	7.1
Dominicans	31.0	30.0	27.8
Cubans	18.0	14.7	16.2
U.S.–born whites	13.0	9.2	5.3

Source.   Reprinted from U.S. Bureau of the Census: "Current Population Reports (Series 3-1)." Washington, DC, U.S. Bureau of the Census, 1993.

their likelihood of receiving health care services, however, increased with their mothers' educational level. The researchers also found that neurotic disorders were more often diagnosed in children of middle-class parents than in children of blue-collar parents and that middle-class children were more likely to be treated with intensive psychotherapy than were children of blue-collar parents. Psychosis or personality disorders were more often diagnosed in children of lower-class parents than in children of middle-class parents. Other authors have also concluded that those in most need received the least service (Ruiz et al. 1995).

■ Acculturation and Acculturative Processes

During the past two decades there has been a surge of interest in the social and psychological impact of acculturation and acculturative stress (Padilla 1980). Contemporary research on acculturation recognizes the variation of immigrant and nonimmigrant minority groups within the national society as well as their influence on the majority population. Contemporary definitions of acculturation now emphasize the changes in social behavior and values between groups that have ongoing contact

TABLE 2. Economic status indicators in total U.S. population and two ethnic minority groups (African Americans and Hispanics)

Ethnic group	Median household income[a]	Below poverty level (%)[a]	Annual income of $50M or more (%)	Home owner- ship (%)[a]	Female-headed households (%)
Total U.S. population	$40,800	11.8	29.0	66.0	16.5
Black Americans	$27,900	23.6	11.9	42.4	47.8
Mexican Americans	$31,950	22.4	11.6	52.7	15.6
Puerto Ricans	$23,080	32.5	11.9	28.3	33.7
Cuban Americans	$36,978	13.5	19.8	57.3	15.3
All Hispanics	$30,700	22.8	14.4	46.1	21.5

[a]Projections by U.S. Bureau of the Census, 1998
Source.   U.S. Bureau of the Census: "Current Population Reports (Series P-20, No. 449)." Washington, DC, U.S. Bureau of the Census, 1991.

with each other (Mavreas et al. 1989). Furthermore, many of the more recent immigrants who have come to the United States as students, business developers, and employees of multinational companies intend to return to their home countries and are committed to retaining their unique cultural characteristics.

A fundamental assumption underlying earlier research on acculturation was that immigrants wished to become assimilated within the larger community and that the host culture actively encouraged such assimilation. This was called the "melting-pot theory" of immigration. This process of acculturative change was viewed as a unidirectional process with immigrant groups losing distinctive aspects of their cultural heritage in favor of "Americanization." In this conceptual framework, people progressed from being unacculturated through the gradients of being minimally, moderately, and fully acculturated. Such unidirectional models of acculturation were experienced by immigrants from war-ravaged Europe to the United States during the first half of the twentieth century. These immigrants often overlooked the prejudice and discrimination within the majority population that limited immigration and strongly resisted immigrants' assimilation.

Today the acculturative process is understood as more interactive, involving acquisition and retention as well as relinquishing in both majority and minority populations (Mavreas et al. 1989; Sodowsky et al. 1991; Szapocznik and Kurtines 1980; Szapocznik et al. 1984). Acculturation is therefore a social process affecting immigrant groups as well as the majority population. The process is envisioned to be continuous over several generations. The rate of change and the circumstances that influence it vary greatly, both between and within groups. For these reasons, studies of groups experiencing acculturative change often divide the groups by temporal experience into first-, second-, and third-generation immigrants. Families within such groups have been categorized as traditional, transitional, or bicultural (Lee 1990). *Traditional* families are characterized as using their native tongues rather than English, living in ethnic enclaves, avoiding interaction with majority cultural institutions, and maintaining preimmigration values and behaviors. *Transitional* families are characterized by greater fluency in the language of the host culture and by children who are becoming familiar with the values and social behaviors of the dominant majority population through attendance at school and school-related activities. *Bicultural* families are defined as those with a high degree of language fluency in their native languages as well as English, economic stability, and residence in multiethnic settings (Lee 1990).

Biculturalism appears to be more adaptive and associated with minimal acculturation stress. Because of this fact, the conceptual and functional aspects of biculturalism have been the focus of much recent research. Scales have been developed to measure the nature and extent of individuals' identification with their cultures of origin and with the majority or host culture (Padilla 1980; Recio Adrados 1993). The Cultural Life Style Inventory (Mendoza 1989) is one such instrument that measures biculturalism. It includes such items as

- Cultural resistance: rejecting the acquisition of new cultural norms while maintaining the original or native ones
- Cultural shift: substituting alternate cultural norms for the native ones
- Cultural incorporation: adapting norms from both cultures

This inventory comprises five domains: intrafamilial language use, extrafamilial language use, social affiliation, cultural familiarity, and cultural identification and pride. The results of studies on the utility of this instrument have led to understanding acculturation in terms of *assimilation,* defined as strong affiliation with the dominant culture; *traditionality,* or rejection of the dominant culture, and *biculturalism,* or ability to assume the behavioral norms of both worlds, with denial of neither (Sodowsky and Plake 1991).

With *bicultural competence,* people can both feel comfortable and function effectively in two distinct cultural contexts (Recio Adrados 1993; Rogler 1989). A more complex issue, understanding the process by which such individuals integrate the elements of both cultural traditions into a psychologically consistent sense of self, remains to be elucidated (Rogler et al. 1991).

Two issues determine the direction of the acculturative process. The first is the extent to which individuals, and the reference group of which they are part, value and wish to preserve their cultural uniqueness, including language, beliefs, values, and behaviors. The second is the extent to which those same individuals and groups value and wish to increase their contact and involvement with other groups, particularly the majority culture. (Note that defining the issues in this way assumes that the majority population is open to and accepting of such increased involvement by a given immigrant or minority population.) The conceptual framework leads to four possible outcomes of acculturative stress (not conceptualized, however, along a unidirectional gradient). The four outcomes are separation, integration, assimilation, and marginalization (Berry 1986; Berry and Kim 1988).

Separation is characterized by individuals' wishes, both conscious and intuitive, to maintain their cultural integrity, 1) by actively resisting the adoption of the values and social behavior patterns of the majority culture or 2) by disengaging themselves from contact with and from the influence of the majority culture. Members of religious cults represent one contemporary example, separatist political movements another.

Integration as an outcome of acculturative stress derives from the desire 1) to maintain a firm sense of original cultural traditions and, at the same time, 2) to incorporate enough of the value system and norms of behavior of the majority culture that group members can feel and behave like members of that culture. The defining feature of integration is therefore a bicultural sense of self, one that intertwines the unique characteristics of two cultural groups. Examples are found among the large numbers of so called "hyphenated Americans," the Italian American, Jewish American, African American, Japanese American, and other people who define their sense of self in terms of their belonging to two cultural traditions. Psychological integration of two cultural traditions is certainly not conflict free; there is continuous intrapsychic struggle to balance inherently conflicting components of a dual identity. That is, the outcome of acculturative stress in any individual is shaped by the particular intrapsychic conflicts and coping abilities of that individual. This phenomenon is what accounts for the great intragroup variation in any population.

Assimilation is the process that results from the conscious and unconscious giving up of the individual's cultural uniqueness in favor of a more or less complete incorporation of the values and behavioral characteristics of another cultural group. Perhaps the most typical examples are those of involuntary assimilation, such that resulting when war and social upheaval motivate or even dictate the changes. Modern examples include individuals from an Eastern European Jewish or an Irish Catholic background who have given up their religion and who attempt to blend in with and identify with the Northern European Protestant majority. However, there are many other situations that motivate people to overlook, suppress, or deny aspects of their cultural heritage and wish to have a seamless fit within another group. As this description suggests, the price, in terms of intrapsychic conflict, can be very high.

Marginalization is another outcome of the rejection or progressive loss of one's cultural heritage, in the context of the values and behavioral norms of the minority cultural group being rejected by the host society. This is an outcome of the acculturative process that is closest to the "identity diffusion" described by Erik Erikson (1968). Identity diffusion is often manifested by the angry, lost, unhappy person who lacks goals and values and whose intense intrapsychic conflicts leave him or her without adequate support systems and at the mercy of much intrafamilial, intergenerational, intracommunity, and intercommunity struggles. Part of their search for psychological meaning and sense of direction is reflected in their turmoil about their ethnic identity.

■ Language

Evaluating language remains one of the most important tasks for the clinician. Language use reflects a wealth of information about the speaker: the clinician can glean insights regarding the patient's origin, education, social class, and intelligence. Clinical assumptions may or may not be accurate and are often influenced by unconsciously held stereotypes (Russell 1988). Thus, when the clinician and the patient do not share language or culture, much information of a cultural nature is obviously lost.

Patients who do not speak a language that the clinician understands pose special problems. Clinicians evaluating patients who do not share their language frequently use interpreters or translators (Kline et al 1980; Sabin 1975; Vasquez and Javier 1991; Westermeyer 1987). Trained interpreters who are accustomed to working with psychiatric patients can be extremely helpful, but they may be unavailable in clinical settings. Thus, the clinician may have to resort for translation purposes to a person who has some knowledge of the patient's language and some knowledge of the clinician's language.

It is crucial to avoid common pitfalls in translations such as distortions, condensations, omissions, and substitutions. The clinician must consider the translator's experience, level of education, relationship to the patient, and relationship to the clinician. These issues may have a profound influence on the quality and accuracy of the translation. For example, a family member is often used to translate for a patient; one can easily envision how this situation could make it difficult for the patient to discuss important matters such as suicidality or sexual problems. Furthermore, a relative may be unwilling to translate material that might be considered embarrassing to the family. In addition, a translator with a low educational level might have difficulty translating some parts of the psychiatric evaluation.

The clinician should encourage the translator to relay what the patient says verbatim. Educating the translator about the symptoms of mental illness can facilitate understanding of material that may sound bizarre or frightening. Topics like suicide, personal finances, or assaultiveness may be sensitive for the translator. In order to maximize rapport with the patient, the clinician should be seated so as to maintain eye contact with the patient; this will enable the clinician to pick up on subtleties of affect and other nonverbal communication. Debriefing the translator afterward also helps the clinician glean as much information as possible from the interview. The sophisticated translator may be able to offer insightful commentary about the patient's language usage, including overinclusiveness, rapidity of speech, and other qualities. A translator from the same culture as the patient can be of further help by translating nonverbal information that may be culturally determined: the translator might be asked about the patient's attire and the meaning of hand or facial gestures. Translators may also render important judgments about the degree to which the patient's experiences or perceptions are culturally syntonic.

Patients who do share a language with the clinician, but not their first language, raise somewhat different questions. Studies of the effect of evaluating severe psychopathology when speaking the patient's second language have had contradictory outcomes (Bamford 1991; Del Castillo 1970; Marcos et al. 1979; Price and Cuellar 1981). Marcos et al. (1979) studied 10 inpatients with schizophrenia who were fluent enough in Spanish and English to respond to items on the Brief Psychiatric Rating Scale (BPRS). These subjects seemed more psychotic when they spoke English than when they spoke Spanish. Yet, when Price and Cuellar (1981) attempted to replicate these findings, subjects seemed more psychotic when speaking Spanish. Thus, the effect of using the first as compared to the second language in evaluations remains obscure. However, Kline et al. (1980) found that patients may feel more understood when interviewed through an interpreter than when interviewed in English, even if the patient is capable of completing the interview in English. In sharp contrast, the clinicians in the Kline et al. study felt that rapport was better when they spoke to the patient directly, without an interpreter.

Bilingual patients may most frequently be unable to express themselves in a second language when acutely psychotic. They may seem withdrawn or have paucity of speech in the second language but be more forthcoming in their mother tongue. This may lead the clinician to an impression of psychosis when the evaluation is conducted in the patient's first language but an impression of psychosis with negative symptomatology in the second. As the patient becomes more organized and able to speak more fluently in the second language, the discrepancy about the perception of negative symptoms may decrease. The evaluation of bilingual patients may also be complicated because the connotations that a word in one language cannot be accurately conveyed by a literal translation. For example, when bilingual patients are interviewed in English, their second language, they may appear perfectly fluent and able to comply with an evaluation yet may unwittingly mislead the clinician. The patient may use an English word accurately but omit its idiomatic or cultural meaning, thus failing to convey possibly crucial information. Ideally, bilingual patients should be evaluated in both languages in order to establish the nature of the psychopathology in each and to unveil eventual discrepancies.

The therapist must also remain alert to cultural issues influencing the use of language in the therapeutic process. Although psychotherapy may be best conducted in the patient's first language, it is not always possible. The therapist should learn about the patient's culture through reading or through consultations with colleagues who have treated patients from that culture. The clinician should also ask the patient about the various cultural domains discussed in this chapter (Cabaniss et al. 1994).

■ Dietary Influences

Although a well-balanced diet is recognized as a requirement for optimal mental health, many areas of the world continue to suffer from endemic nutritional deficiencies (Desjarlais et al. 1995). It has been well documented that dietary deficiencies increase the tendency to develop a variety of acute and chronic illnesses (including mental illnesses) and can also promote developmental abnormalities. Although public health initiatives have significantly reduced the prevalence of mental illness secondary to nutritional deficiency in the United States compared with the prevalence a century ago, suboptimal nutritional patterns persist in many rural and urban areas. Particularly at risk for illnesses induced by nutritional deficiency are pockets of population in which the ethnocultural milieu is (voluntarily or involuntarily) far removed from the mainstream culture, often as a result of either poor financial means or limited education. The clinical index of suspicion for psychiatric symptomatology secondary to nutritional deficiency should be high when evaluating individuals from impoverished areas or recent immigrants with unknown or significantly different dietary backgrounds. For example, one of the first proven etiologies of a nutritionally acquired illness with dramatic psychopathology was the demonstration in the United States early this century that the symptomatic triad of depression/dementia, dermatitis, and diarrhea of pellagra was due to a deficiency of the B vitamin niacin. Such dietary deficiencies can easily occur in individuals whose diet consists largely of maize, as has been common historically in certain agrarian groups.

Nutritional deficiency associated with mental illness is not limited to immigrants or to impoverished members of society. Anorexia nervosa and bulimia occur primarily among girls and young women from relatively wealthy, "first-world" countries whose culturally based ideals of body image and beauty promote severe food restriction in order to achieve fashion-runway, model-slim figures. Heretofore uncommon outside the United States and Europe, anorexia nervosa and bulimia are now being seen with greater frequency in Japan and countries of Southeast Asia as Western cultural values are rapidly spread via commerce and mass media. In the mid-1990s, the world of high fashion increased the cultural cachet of severe food restriction with the glorification of an emaciated, waiflike look embodied by the so-called supermodels. Unfortunately, these culturally based eating disorders may be physiologically self-reinforcing on a neuroendocrine level, because both the severe food restriction of anorexia nervosa and the repetitive binge-purge activity of bulimia can produce euphoria secondary to the release of endogenous opiates.

In other cultural situations, the inclusion of certain plants, animals, and minerals in the diet can have dramatic intentional or unintentional neuropsychiatric effects. Throughout Europe during the Middle Ages, stored grains (particularly barley and rye) sometimes became infected with the ergot fungus and caused sporadic outbreaks of toxic hallucinatory psychoses and occasional fatalities in the general population. They are also believed to have been a significant contributor to mental illness and the cause of thousands of deaths in several epidemic poisonings. In several cultures throughout recorded history, certain ingredients used specifically for food preparation or preservation have not only served to stimulate the palate, but have also frequently been used for their psychotropic effects. For example, anthropologists have described communal eating ceremonies preceding religious spiritual trances or in preparation for battle, much as alcohol accompanying a meal is frequently used to loosen inhibitions or prohibitions. It has also been well documented that the purposeful consumption, in both eating and drinking, of hallucinogenic plants has played important cultural roles in diverse civilizations over thousands of years. Examination of scenes represented in several kinds of domestic artifacts or utensils has led to the conclusion that, in antiquity, dramatic alterations in perception and behavior, resulting from diets containing hallucinogenic plants, not only promoted differences between ethnocultural groups but probably contributed to the evolution of spirituality and religion through the sharing of transcendental ego-dissolving, psychedelic experiences. In many cultures, explanatory models of illness often favor the use of herbal medicines, vitamins, and food over traditional pharmacotherapy (Jacobsen and Comas-Diaz 1999).

The 1976 Nobel Prize in Medicine was awarded for the finding that a fatal neurodegenerative illness called *kuru* was transmitted by the ingestion of an infectious neurogenetic agent called a prion. The research demonstrated the interaction of culture, diet, and neuropsychiatric illness: the transmission of this deadly slow virus occurred primarily in cannibals of the Fore tribe of Papua New Guinea, whose diet included the ritual consumption of human brains. Another recent example demonstrates that cultural influences on diet in the spread of neuropsychiatric pathology are not limited to ancient times or to isolated indigenous populations. In England, the time-honored cultural tradition of heavy meat consumption (popularly illustrated by the "Beefeater" figure) led in the mid-1990s to a number of cases of the fatal dementing illness dubbed "mad cow disease." Cows and sheep have long been recognized as being subject to sporadic outbreaks of a fatal neurodegenerative illness called scrapie which, like *kuru,* results from a prion infection of the central nervous system (Emson et al. 1993). The penny-pinching agricultural practice of pulverizing an entire cow's (or sheep's) body for inclusion in animal feed (which has also been practiced in some areas of the United States) led to a cross-species contagion when prion-infected beef was consumed by humans. (Unfortunately, prions are not killed by conventional cooking techniques.) England was forced by a European and United States boycott to destroy its entire beef supply for over a year and has now reportedly eliminated infectious feeding practices, but the often considerable time delay in neuropsychiatric presentation of slow viruses unfortunately suggests that latent cases of people infected with mad cow disease may not become manifest for many years into the future. Finally, in an example of a cultural trend toward consumption of nontraditional or natural substances for health, unregulated over-the-counter sales of the so-called natural sleeping pill melatonin have continued unabated in the United States and abroad, even though a major source of melatonin has historically been the pineal glands of sheep, which can also carry the infectious prions.

Ethnocultural dietary influences can have dramatic effects on the pharmacology of both psychotropic and nonpsychotropic medications by changing their absorption, metabolism, distribution, and elimination. These pharmacological influences depend on individual and familial genetic inheritance as well as on interaction with specific factors in the environment. For example, advances in the understanding of drug metabolism have revealed that genetically controlled liver enzyme systems (particularly the cytochrome P450 system) can show substantial racial/ethnic variation in both the amount and in the activity of enzymes that metabolize many common medications, including psychotropics. If a cytochrome enzyme responsible for the metabolism of a particular psychotropic has diminished activity (or is missing), toxic levels of the drug may occur. For example, African Americans and Southeast Asians have been found in some studies to require lower doses of tricyclic antidepressants than do Caucasians to attain therapeutic responses and to avoid toxicity. Unfortunately, the vast majority of psychopharmacological trials not only fail to take such ethnic variations into consideration but frequently fail even to report the ethnic composition of their subjects. This problem has been further compounded until quite recently by the exclusion of women from many pharmacologic trials (Lin et al. 1993).

Ethnoculturally determined pharmacological influences can occur as a result of differences in food composition, preparation, and even the circadian timing of feeding. Studies in England, for example, have found that among both Sudanese and Asian Indian immigrants, individuals who maintain their native vegetarian diets tend to have profiles of cytochrome P450 enzyme activity different from that of immigrants who adopt the mainstream British meat-eating diet (Jacobsen 1994). Throughout much of Latin America the *hot and cold theory* dictates that foods culturally characterized as hot should not be consumed concurrently with foods characterized as cold, thereby leading to variations in food intake that could conceivably alter pharmacologic (and behavioral) activity.

Most published reports investigating the pharmacologic implications of ethnoculturally determined dietary influences have tended to concentrate on dramatic toxic reactions such as the so-called "Chinese restaurant syndrome," an uncomfortable and occasionally severe neurovascular flushing caused by the ingestion of food prepared with the addition of monosodium glutamate, a flavor-enhancing excitatory neurotransmitter. In the realm of everyday psychopharmacologic practice, the surging popularity of the so-called Mediterranean diet has been associated with an increase in the number of people consuming dishes containing fava beans. These beans, because of a high content of the neurotransmitter dopamine, can cause severe hypertensive reactions in individuals taking monoamine oxidase inhibitors (MAOIs). More recently, grapefruit juice has been found to inhibit the cytochrome P450 3A4 isozyme, which is responsible for metabolizing a number of psychotropics, including sertraline, nefazodone, trazodone, fluoxetine, buspirone, and numerous benzodiazepines (as well as many nonpsychotropic medications). Consuming the juice can therefore cause dramatic elevations in the blood levels of these drugs. The importance of such interactive effects is underscored by the fact that deaths have occurred when some of these medications have been taken concurrently with the 3A4-metabolized antihistamines terfenadine (Seldane) and astemizole (Hismanal), by interfering with the metabolism of the antihistamines and thereby elevating their blood levels into a fatally cardiotoxic range. (In fact, Hismanal and terfenadine-containing medications were withdrawn from the market in the United States in the late 1990s.)

The communal act of eating is perhaps the most frequently occurring family or group behavior in many ethnocultural groups. Communal meals provide a public or semipublic stage where latent psychopathology may be first manifested, for example, through refusal of food, refusal to partake in communal eating, or unusual feeding behavior. Food-related behavior is often assessed by the family and community as a basic indicator of social acceptability, and cultural patterns have evolved in most societies to carefully regulate communal feeding behaviors (McKenna 1992). Parental injunctions such as "Don't play with your food!" have cultural as well as socioeconomic implications and carry greater mental health implications than often assumed (COSSMHO 1988). Individual abnormalities in eating behaviors such as bulimia have developed primarily in societies in which the relative abundance of food causes the pattern of adult diet to be more reflective of creating an individual's social image than of achieving minimal nutritional requirements, whereas such psychopathology is predictably less common in sociocultural groups in which food is scarce.

Environmental factors such as geography, climate, and the fertility of the land also contribute to ethnoculturally determined dietary patterns and their related psychopathologies. For example, epidemiological studies in North America found that, in areas subject to increasingly severe seasonal changes, individuals show correspondingly higher rates of seasonal affective disorder, and in addition the nonaffectively ill population shows increasing rates of fall/winter problems, such as carbohydrate craving and weight gain. Environmentally induced exacerbation of ethnoculturally related psychopathology (such as bulimia) may thereby be greater in more northerly climates (Porges 1997; Sapolsky 1997).

■ Education

The initial interaction of patient and psychiatrist is central to eliciting information that will lead to the formulation of a diagnosis or a treatment plan. Although other factors, such as race and gender, obviously play a role in this interaction, education may influence the outcome of the interview by having an impact on both the language and the nonverbal communication used by both the patient and the clinician (Leininger 1984). Education may also exert a positive influence on patients as they try to respond to the physician's questions about the nature and duration of the complaint as well as about what factors exacerbate it. Insofar as an articulate presentation of one's pain and suffering is a function of education, it also influences the facility and rapidity of the connection between the patient and the mental health clinician. Obviously, education may also enhance the patients' presentations of their treatment histories, concurrent medical conditions, and medications they are taking at the time of the evaluation. Being educated should also make it easier for patients to describe other complicated aspects of their backgrounds, such as sexual history.

Poor education may sometimes complicate the establishment of a positive and interactive relationship between patient and psychiatrist, especially in situations where the patient's deficient education is exaggerated by an unfamiliar regional accent or generally poor linguistic expression. The situation is of course worsened by a patient's personal shyness or characterological reticence. Russell (1988) has reminded us that education, particularly as mediated through language, may have both positive and negative effects on the psychotherapeutic relationship. In conjunction with socioeconomic status, it may influence patients' perceptions of an illness and its etiological basis. One's educational level may also have some impact on symptom expression and on one's willingness to attribute symptomatic complaints to psychological as opposed to organic or somatic origins. The potential impact of education on the diagnostic assessment and the mental status examination is another area of concern (Tseng and McDermott 1981; Eisenberg 1988). Tests of abstract thinking usually focus on similarities, differences, and the meaning of proverbs. Such questions may simply make no sense to the poorly educated patient. Consequently, concrete or incorrect responses from the poorly educated should not be taken to mean serious psychopathology in every case. Tests of concentration such as serial 7s are often too difficult with patients whose educational level is minimal, and an easier standard should be applied, such as subtracting 3 from 20. Equal care should be taken with the use of tests like recalling digits backwards and forwards. Although the average patient may be at ease with such testing techniques, the poorly educated patient may be panicked by such requirements in the course of an encounter with a health professional.

The examination of the poorly educated patient requires patience and willingness on the clinician's part to help the patient relax. The clinician should also make an effort to gauge the patient's capacity to think abstractly and to concentrate through discussion of activities that are more readily familiar to the patient. For example, even poorly educated patients may have a passion for a particular sport like basketball. The patient may be able to explain quite sophisticated strategies for winning a game. Patients often give surprising details of who the players are on a specific team and may analyze quite effectively the strengths and weaknesses of the team. Such unorthodox approaches to the poorly educated patient may provide enough information to help the clinician avoid confusing psychopathology with behavioral styles, language, and thinking rooted in deficient education.

Education, especially when intermingled with other cultural elements, has been noted to have significant impact on the results of standardized psychological tests, particularly intelligence tests (Williams 1987). This has caused considerable debate in the past; some workers have argued that the standardization of intelligence tests works consistently to the disadvantage of groups who have not been educated in the same way as have the dominant groups. Clinicians should therefore be cautious in their interpretations of and conclusions extracted from the results.

■ References

Adebimpe VR: Overview: white norms and psychiatric diagnosis of black patients. Am J Psychiatry 138:279–285, 1981

American Psychiatric Association: Ethnic Minority Elderly. Washington, DC, American Psychiatric Press, 1994

American Psychiatric Association: Diagnostic and Statistical Manual of Mental Disorders, 4th Edition, Text Revision. Washington, DC, American Psychiatric Association, 2000

Astrachan A: How Men Feel. New York, Anchor Press/Doubleday, 1988

Bamford K: Bilingual issues in mental health assessment and treatment. Hispanic Journal of Behavioral Sciences 12:377–390, 1991

Berry JW: The acculturation process and refugee behavior, in Refugee Mental Health in Resettlement Countries. Edited by CL Williams, J Westermeyer. New York, Hemisphere Press, 1986, pp 138–152

Berry JW, Kim U: Acculturation and mental health, in Health and Cross-Cultural Psychology: Toward Applications. Edited by Dasen P, Berry JW, Sartorius N. Newbury Park, CA, Sage, 1988, pp 114–122

Bland IJ: Adolescent girl to woman: developmental issues in transition. Louisiana Psychiatric Association Newsletter 29, Winter 1994, p 2

Bradshaw WH Jr: Supervision in black and white: race as a factor in supervision, in Applied Supervision in Psychotherapy. Edited by Blumenfield M. New York, Grune & Stratton, 1982, pp 213–219

Browning DS, Jobe T, Evison IS (eds): Religious and Ethical Factors in Psychiatric Practice. Chicago, Nelson-Hall, 1990

Brumberg JJ: Fasting Girls: The History of Anorexia Nervosa. New York, New American Library, 1989

Burton LA (ed): Religion and the Family. New York, Haworth, 1992

Cabaniss D, Oquendo M, Singer M: The impact of psychoanalytic values on transference and counter-transference: a study in transcultural psychotherapy. Journal of the Academy of Psychoanalysis 22(4):609–622, 1994

Canino I, Spurlock J (eds): Culturally Diverse Children and Adolescents. New York, Guilford, 1994

Clower VL: The acquisition of mature femininity, in Women and Men. Edited by Notman M, Nadelson C. Washington, DC, American Psychiatric Press, 1991, pp 75–88

Comas-Diaz L, Greene B (eds): Women of Color. New York, Guilford, 1994

Comas-Diaz L, Jacobsen FM: Ethnocultural transference and countertransference in the therapeutic dyad. Am J Orthopsychiatry 61:392–402, 1991

COSSMHO: Delivering Preventive Health Care to Hispanics: A Manual for Providers. Washington, DC, The National Coalition of Hispanic Health and Human Services Organizations, 1988

Cross W: Shades of Black. Philadelphia, PA, Temple University Press, 1991

Del Castillo JC: The influence of language upon symptomatology in foreign-born patients. Am J Psychiatry 127:242–244, 1970

Desjarlais R, Eisenberg L, Good B, et al: World Mental Health: Problems and Priorities in Low-Income Countries. New York, Oxford University Press, 1995

Dohrenwend BP, Dohrenwend BS, Gould MS, et al: Mental Illness in the United States. New York, Praeger, 1980

Eisenberg L: The social construction of mental illness. Psychol Med 18(1):1–9, 1988

Emson PC, Augood SJ, Senaris R, et al: Chemical signaling and striatal interneurons. Prog Brain Res 99:155–165, 1993

Erikson EH: Identity, Youth and Crisis. New York, Norton, 1968

Fabrega H Jr, Ulrich R, Mezzich JE: Do Caucasian and black adolescents differ at psychiatric intake? J Am Acad Child Adolesc Psychiatry 32:407–413, 1993

Flaskerud JH, Hu JL: Relationship of ethnicity to psychiatric diagnosis. J Nerv Ment Dis 180:296–303, 1992

Fried M: Disadvantage, vulnerability, and mental health, in Behavior, Health Risks and Social Disadvantage. Edited by Parron D, Solomon F, Jenkins C. Washington, DC, National Academy Press, 1982, pp 42–52

Fullilove MT: Minority women: ecological setting and intercultural dialogue, in Psychological Aspects of Women's Health Care. Edited by Stewart D, Stotland N. Washington, DC, American Psychiatric Press, 1993, pp 519–539

Gaines A: Ethnopsychiatry. Honolulu, HI, University of Hawaii Press, 1991

Gaw AC: Psychiatric care of Chinese Americans, in Culture, Ethnicity and Mental Illness. Edited by Gaw A. Washington, DC, American Psychiatric Press, 1993, pp 245–280

Grier WH, Cobbs P: Black Rage. New York, Bantam Books, 1968

Griffith E, Young J: A cross-cultural introduction to the therapeutic aspect of Christian religious ritual, in Clinical Guidelines in Cross-Cultural Mental Health. Edited by Comas-Diaz L, Griffith E. New York, Wiley, 1988, pp 89–94

Jacobsen FM: Psychopharmacology, in Women of Color: Integrating Ethnic and Gender Identities in Psychotherapy. Edited by Comas-Diaz L, Greene B. New York, Guilford, 1994, pp 319–338

Jacobsen FM, Comas-Diaz L: Psychopharmacological Treatment of Latinas. Essential Psychopharmacology 3:29–42, 1999

Jones BE, Gray BA: Problems in diagnosing schizophrenia and affective disorders among blacks. Hospital and Community Psychiatry 37:61–65, 1986

Karno M, Hough RL, Burnam A, et al: Lifetime prevalence of specific psychiatric disorders among Mexican Americans and non-Hispanic whites in Los Angeles. Arch Gen Psychiatry 44:695–701, 1987

Kelly G: The Psychology of Personal Constructs, Vols 1 and 2. New York, WW Norton, 1955

Kirmayer LJ: Cultural variations in the response to psychiatric disorders and emotional distress. Soc Sci Med 29:327–339, 1989

Kleinman A: Rethinking Psychiatry. New York, Free Press, 1988

Kline F, Acosta FX, Austin W, et al: The misunderstood Spanish-speaking patient. Am J Psychiatry 137:1530–1533, 1980

Kluckhohn C: Navaho Witchcraft. Boston, MA, Beacon Press, 1967

Langner TS, Gersten J, Eisenberg J: Approaches to measurement and definition in the epidemiology of behavior disorders: ethnic background and child behavior. Int J Health Serv 4:483–501, 1974

Larson D: The Faith Factor: An Annotated Bibliography of Systematic Reviews and Clinical Research on Spiritual Subjects (Vol 2). Rockville, MD, National Institute for Healthcare Research, 1993

Last CG, Perrin S: Anxiety and disorders in African-American and white children. J Abnorm Child Psychol 21:153–164, 1993

Lee E: Assessment and treatment of Chinese-American immigrant families, in Minorities and Family Therapy. Edited by Saba G, Karrer B, Hardy K. New York, Haworth, 1990, pp 191–209

Leininger M: Transcultural interviewing and health assessment, in Mental Health Services: The Cross-Cultural Contest. Edited by Pedersen PB, Sartorius N, Marsella AJ. Beverly Hills, CA, Sage, 1984, pp 112–118

Lin TY, Lin MC: Love, denial, and rejection: responses of Chinese families to mental illness, in Normal and Abnormal Behavior in Chinese Culture. Edited by Kleinman A, Lin T. Dordrecht, Netherlands, Reidel, 1981, pp 135–142

Lin KM, Poland RE, Silver B: Overview: the interface between psychobiology and ethnicity, in Psychopharmacology and Psychobiology of Ethnicity. Edited by Lin KM, Poland RE, Nakasaki G. Washington, DC, American Psychiatric Press, 1993, pp 11–35

Littlewood R: An indigenous conceptualization of reactive depression in Trinidad. Psychol Med 15:275–280, 1985

Lukoff D, Lu F, Turner R: Toward a more culturally sensitive DSM-IV: psychoreligious and psychospiritual problems. J Nerv Ment Dis 180:673–682, 1992

Lukoff D, Turner R, Lu F: Transpersonal psychology research review: psychoreligious dimensions of healing. Journal of Transpersonal Psychology 24:41–60, 1992

Lukoff D, Turner R, Lu F: Transpersonal psychology research review: psychospiritual dimensions of healing. Journal of Transpersonal Psychology 25:11–28, 1993

Madsen W: Mexican-Americans of South Texas. New York, Holt, Rinehart and Winston, 1973

Mahler MS, Pine F, Bergman A: The Psychological Birth of the Human Infant: Symbiosis and Individuation. New York, Basic Books, 1975

Marcos LR, Uruyo L, Kesselman M, et al: The language barrier in evaluating Spanish-American patients. Arch Gen Psychiatry 29:655–659, 1979

Mavreas V, Bebbington P, Der G: The structure and validity of acculturative: analysis of an acculturative scale. Social Psychiatry and Epidemiology 24: 233–240, 1989

McGoldrick M, Pearce JK, Giordano J (eds): Ethnicity and Family Therapy. New York, Guilford, 1982

McKenna T: Food of the Gods. New York, Bantam Books, 1992

Mendoza RH: An empirical scale to measure type and degree of acculturation in Mexican American adolescents and adults. Journal of Cross-Cultural Psychology 20:372–385, 1989

Merrill WL: Raramuri: Souls, Knowledge and Social Process in Northern Mexico. Washington, DC, Smithsonian Institution Press, 1988

Moore BE, Fine BD: Psychoanalytic Terms and Concepts. New Haven, CT, The American Psychoanalytic Association and Yale University Press, 1990

Newhill CE: The role of culture in the development of paranoid symptomatology. Am J Orthopsychiatry 60:176–185, 1990

Notman MT, Nadelson CC: Women and Men: New Perspectives on Gender Differences. Washington, DC, American Psychiatric Press, 1991

Padilla AM: The role of cultural awareness and ethnic loyalty in acculturation, in Acculturation: Theory, Models and Some New Findings. Edited by Padilla AM. Boulder, CO, Westview Press, 1980, pp 27–44

Pedersen P, Ivey A: Culture-Centered Counseling and Interviewing Skills. Westport, CT, Praeger, 1993

Porges SW: Emotion: an evolutionary by-product of the neural regulation of the autonomic nervous system. Ann N Y Acad Sci 807:62–77, 1997

Price C, Cuellar I: Effects of language and related variables on the expression of psychotherapy in Mexican American Psychiatric patients. Hispanic Journal of the Behavioral Sciences 3:145–160, 1981

Recio Adrados JL: Acculturation: the broader view: theoretical framework of the acculturation scales, in Drug Abuse Among Minority Youth: Advances in Research and Methodology. Edited by De La Rosa MR, Recio Adrados JL. NIDA Research Monograph. Washington, DC, National Institute on Drug Abuse, 1993, pp 15–24

Rogler LH: The meaning of culturally sensitive research in mental health. Am J Psychiatry 166:296–303, 1989

Rogler LH, Cortés DE: Help-seeking pathways: a unifying concept in mental health care. Am J Psychiatry 150:554–561, 1993

Rogler LH, Cortés DE, Malgady RG: Acculturation and mental health status among Hispanics: convergence and new directions for research. Am Psychol 45:585–597, 1991

Ruiz P, Venegas K, Alarcón RD: the economics of pain: mental health care costs among minorities. Psychiatr Clin North Am 18:659–670, 1995

Russell DM: Language and psychotherapy. the influence of non-standard English in clinical practice, in Clinical Guidelines in Cross-Cultural Mental Health. Edited by Comas-Diaz L, Griffith EEH. New York, Wiley, 1988

Sabin JE: Translating despair. Am J Psychiatry 132:197–199, 1975

Sakauye K: The elderly Asian patient. Am J Geriatr Psychiatry 25:85–104, 1992

Sapolsky RM: The Trouble with Testosterone. New York, Scribner, 1997

Sodowsky GR, Plake BS: Psychometric properties of the American-International relations scale. Educational and Psychological Measurement 51: 207–217, 1991

Sodowsky GR, Lai EWM, Plake BS: Moderating effects of sociocultural variables on acculturation attributes of Hispanics and Asian Americans. Journal of Counseling and Development 70:194–204, 1991

Stein TS: Changing perspectives on homosexuality, in American Psychiatric Press Review of Psychiatry, Vol 12. Edited by Oldham J, Riba M, Tasman A. Washington, DC, American Psychiatric Press, 1993, pp 3–129

Stoller RJ: Sex and Gender: On The Development of Masculinity and Femininity. New York, Science House, 1968

Sue D, Arredondo P, McDavis RJ: Multi-cultural counseling competencies and standards. Journal of Counseling and Development 10:447–486, 1992

Szapocznik J, Kurtines WZ: Acculturation, biculturalism and adjustment among Cuban Americans, in Acculturation: Theory, Models, and Some New Findings. Edited by Padilla AM. Boulder, CO, Westview Press, 1980, pp 139–159

Szapocznik J, Santisteban D, Kurtines W, et al: Bicultural effectiveness training: a treatment intervention for enhancing intercultural adjustment in Cuban American families. Hispanic Journal of Behavioral Science 6: 317–344, 1984

Tseng W-S, McDermott JF: Culture, Mind and Therapy: An Introduction to Cultural Psychiatry. New York, Brunner/Mazel, 1981

U.S. Bureau of the Census: Current Population Reports. Series P-20, No. 449. Washington, DC, U.S. Government Printing Office, 1991

U.S. Bureau of the Census: The Foreign Born Population in the United States. Current Population Reports, Series 3-1. Washington, DC, U.S. Government Printing Office, 1993

Vasquez C, Javier RA: The problem with interpreters: communicating with Spanish-speaking patients. Hospital and Community Psychiatry 42:163–165, 1991

Westermeyer J: Clinical considerations in cross-cultural diagnosis. Hospital and Community Psychiatry 38:160–165, 1987

Westermeyer JJ: Cross-cultural psychiatric assessment, in Culture, Ethnicity, and Mental Illness. Edited by Gaw A. Washington, DC, American Psychiatric Press, 1993, pp 125–144

Williams CL: Issues surrounding psychological testing of minority patients. Hospital and Community Psychiatry 38:184–189, 1987

Yamamoto J: Japanese Americans, in Cross-Cultural Psychiatry. Boston, MA, John Wright, 1982

3

Cultural Formulation: Description and Clinical Use

Case formulations elaborate on a given diagnosis to facilitate the understanding of the patient's plight. In doing so, they go from the broad, categorical description to the particular, personalized perspective of the story. Mezzich (1995) calls case formulations idiographic statements intended "to supplement standardized diagnostic ratings with a narrative description of the cultural framework of the patient's identity, illness, and social context, and of the clinician-patient relationship" (p. 649). Identifying data are a first step in this process of particularization—an epidemiological template based on features such as age, gender, family history, race, language, and lifestyle. A multiaxial diagnostic system also moves from the general to the more particular, accounting for comorbidities, severity of stress, and level of functioning. This movement leads to further distillation of the case into smaller classes. An approach that elaborates on unique features of the patient's developmental history has been a cornerstone of the psychodynamic formulation, guided by psychoanalytical precepts (Gedo and Goldberg 1973). Thus, a formulation is a detailed elaboration and substantiation of the diagnosis, a justification of its pertinence and value. In this chapter we examine characteristics that, originating from the patient's membership in a given culture, confer special meaning and shape on his or her clinical manifestations and help to establish a comprehensive case formulation.

The foregoing also allows the conceptualization of a case formulation as a therapeutic first step. As the development of treatment guidelines and clinical pathways demonstrates (American Psychiatric Association 2000), a diagnosis of a clinical entity has treatment implications rooted in its pathophysiology and pathogenesis. The emphasis on individualized treatment plans in accreditation standards reflects attempts to solve the dilemma posed by the lack of treatment specificity for broad diagnostic categories. It follows that the more particular the definition of a clinical state, the more specific the therapeutic interventions become. Matching treatment to diagnosis is increasingly visualized through a case study method that relies on a formulation (Nurcombe and Gallagher 1986). The classical psychodynamic formulation was certainly an attempt at initiating a well-thought-out therapeutic plan—that is, a conception of pathogenesis and subsequent treatment interventions that focused on the particulars of an individual patient's life history.

A cultural formulation, the subject of this chapter, contributes not only to refining the epidemiological particularities of the case but also to a careful examination of dimensions that give meaning to a patient's experience and ultimately facilitate treatment. No other medical specialty makes the meaning of an experience, pathological or otherwise, central to its enterprise as psychiatry does. Yet the idea of a cultural formulation as a formal part of the diagnostic assessment is relatively recent (Fabrega 1996). In what became a classic in the training of psychiatrists in the United States, the so-called Menninger Manual, Karl Menninger (1962) presented a format for a case formulation. Although the emphasis was on the psychodynamic aspects of the clinical history, various cultural characteristics of a patient (philosophical, social, and religious) were to be explored and described in the narrative. The cultural formulation, as contemporaneously conceived, adds several important factors to the general case formulation. It allows the clinician a framework for understanding the patient's cultural identity, cultural explanation of illness, cultural factors in the psychosocial environment, and cultural elements of the relationship between patient and clinician.

The need for explaining a patient's cultural background and accounting for it in a total understanding of his or her situation has become generally accepted only in recent years. The era of cataloging esoteric "culture-bound syndromes" has given way to a more subtle appreciation of the psychosocial implications of a person's culture in clinical occurrences. Not only has the literature on cross-cultural and transcultural comparisons abounded; a more systematic and sympathetic exploration of all cultures (including those of the Western world) and their relationship to mental health and illness has become widely feasible. The presence of minority and immigrant populations from heterogeneous cultures in the United States, among both patients and clinicians, has certainly given impetus to this trend, as documented by their demands to count and to be understood—in and on their own terms. During the developmental phase of DSM-IV, leading cultural psychiatrists (Good 1996; Kleinman 1988) posed the challenge of including a cultural axis and settled on the elaboration of a cultural formulation included in DSM-IV's Appendix I. The history of these efforts is well documented in the literature (Alarcón 1995; Kleinman 1996; Mezzich et al. 1993).

■ The DSM-IV-TR Model

The outline in DSM-IV-TR (American Psychiatric Association 2000; this is the latest version of DSM-IV) proposes four major themes and an overall assessment of patients in considering a cultural formulation (see Appendix I in DSM-IV-TR for a full text of the cultural formulation guidelines). In this section we analyze the nature and content of each of these components, stressing both their theoretical and practical characteristics.

Cultural Identity of the Patient

Identity implies uniqueness, a set of special features coming together to form a whole. Cultural identity implies the characteristics shared by a group, a person's culture. Thus identity allows for a self-definition, involving self-esteem, special skills and talents, role in work and family, and place in the social order. This idea has been largely shaped by the work of Erikson (1950, 1959), who, although looking for epigenetic universals in the life cycle, nevertheless focused on critical pathways in the development of various cultural groups.

Of the several variables that contribute to the construction of an identity, as seen in Chapter 2, membership in a particular group (ethnic, racial, national, or of any other kind) plays a significant part. Ultimately, culture defines what it means to be a person—who one is, by what values one is governed, what is sacred and what is profane, who others are, and in what relationship level one stands to them. For example: Is marriage a contract or a covenant? and hence, What is the meaning of divorce? Is the acceptance of parental authority a sign of dependence or a moral obligation? and hence, What is the meaning of obedience and self-assertion? Such questions are obviously oversimplified and appear rhetorical, since individuals and groups may attach various degrees of relevance to the values implicit in them. Clinicians are becoming familiar with cultural variations in sexuality and gender roles and must also come to appreciate other orders of cultural difference such as hierarchies of age, rank and status, and family configurations.

Shweder and Bourne (1982) have suggested that the concept of the person varies across cultures. They identify two major alternative types of personal organizations, which they term "egocentric-contractual" (individualistic, subjected to and limited by sociocultural rules) and "sociocentric-organic" (outward-directed, closely integrated with the surrounding environment). Various other distinctions and perspectives exist: achievement orientation and affiliation orientation, self-directed and other-directed or field dependent. All of them have somewhat similar meanings and attempt to highlight contrasts between personality types and styles of cultural adaptation. Sampson (1988) and many others have argued that individualism is more an indigenous Western philosophical and practical principle than a universally espoused standard of social life and mental health. The one fundamental point at which these different conceptualizations converge is that the notion of identity is constrained by the boundaries of one's skin and that the idea of complete autonomy is ultimately a Western psychological and cultural myth (Desai and Collins 1985). In any transaction, dyadic or otherwise, assumptions about how separate one is from the other, or whether one is autonomous or part of a group, determine the nature of the transaction (Marriott 1990).

Categorizing cultures along any of these dimensions may appear like stereotyping. Yet not all individuals adhere to group norms to the same degree or with the same intensity. Careful evaluation of a person's investment in and identification with a group—or, conversely, how alienated from the group the person is or how defensive the cultural armor may have become—obviates the danger of prejudice and prejudgment. However, it is paramount not to regard values and ideals as merely peripheral or derivative, because culturally based developmental influences shape the very nature of self in action.

The problem of differentiation within a cultural group is further complicated by geographic mobility, industrialization, urbanization, biracial marriages, and immigration. Socioeconomic and political forces are also reshaping the lifestyles of ethnic groups and may usher in a variety of adaptations or maladaptations, including alienation and anomie (Durkheim 1951). Social change brought about by moving to a different culture may require mapping the trajectory of the identified person as well as his or her group, and an examination of the cultural distance between the guest and the host and of strategies for coping with an alien culture (Desai and Coehlo 1986). It is important to remember that to acclimate is not necessarily to acculturate, and strategies that worked earlier in life may produce degrees of maladaptation in the new situation. Attempts at immersion in the host culture and consequent assimilation are no different, in terms of their nature and the amount of inner effort and stress involved, than is remaining bound to the old culture. Metaphors like *melting pot* or *mosaic* must be distilled down to cohesion and continuity of identity. Undoubtedly, the rich information these sources provide for the clinical history of a patient is an invaluable component in the understanding of the case, and of the patient as a person.

Cultural Explanation of the Illness

In the era of alternative medicine, Americans have become familiar with apothecaries of other cultures, herbal medicine, acupuncture, and the practice of meditation and yoga. What is less recognized is that below the surface of these cultural invasions are elaborate concepts of body construction and vastly different notions of pathophysiology and pathogenesis. This is particularly so for disorders such as mental illnesses, in which dimensions beyond the physical may be involved. Complex demonological explanations, spirit possession, "evil eye," and "soul loss" are some of the models of mental illness among various cultures of the world. More systematized medical models based on humoral theories and energy distribution with attendant pathophysiology are not uncommon. Models based on trauma and injury at the physical level, shock, insults, jealousy, "nerves," and exhaustion also abound. Predispositions may be explained in various cultures by body type, familial genetic loading, biochemical imbalances, astrological influences, sinfulness, or *karma*. Thus, asking patients about their unique explanatory models of illness (Kleinman 1988) and about their conceptions of the cause and roots of their clinical symptoms opens up revealing pathways into their cultural world and their most intimate fears, hopes, anxieties, and emotions. Similarly, clarifying the meaning of an illness to patients, with clear respect for their own notions, may facilitate trust, communication, and the sharing of therapeutic strategies. This does not mean that a therapist has to abandon his or her own paradigm, since a path to a renewed exploration of the illness may suggest itself.

Another important dimension of cultural explanations is that of idioms of distress. Nichter (1981) clarified the ways in which patients may articulate their experience of illness and at the same time evoke a response from caregivers who understand the help-seeking behavior as a shared means of communication. Kleinman (1977) demonstrated that among Chinese populations, depression manifests itself with somatic symptoms—"somatization." This is not unlike what happens in many developing countries and predominantly agrarian cultures. Kakar (1982) has dealt sensitively with the issue of idioms of distress in India. The basic value of these idioms in the clinical endeavor is the conveying of a message that reflects—mostly under the guise of a socially accepted complaint or ailment—deeply felt individual or collective suffering. Culturally aware clinicians can use this knowledge to immerse themselves in the patient's repertoire of symbols and to help in the understanding and management of the presenting symptoms.

Cultural Factors Related to the Psychosocial Environment of the Patient

This has to do primarily with the kind, strength, scope, and consistency of the so-called support systems. Obviously, there are cultural variations in each patient's psychosocial environment, and a cultural perspective is both narrower than the psychosocial and different from it, in spite of the many connections between the two. The cultural aspects of this environment entail dealing not only with issues such as physical proximity but also with how kin networks provide emotional, instrumental, and informational support and with how that can be articulated into diagnostic and therapeutic efforts (McGoldrick et al. 1996). Key among social support components are those of a religious and spiritual nature (Lukoff et al. 1995). The ritualistic (symbolic) nature of these beliefs and their practices strengthens the inner recovery forces that result from culturally infused values, norms and principles regarding adversity, human flaws, failure, or conflict. They also allow the clinician-therapist to reinforce the sense of self-respect the patient needs in order to restore self-esteem and the desire to go on. Needless to say, iatrogenesis is a risk in the assessment and management of these issues; on the other hand, its successful handling has a positive effect on the outcome.

A concern about cultural perspectives in the psychosocial environment of the patient stems from what are regarded as givens in the West, especially the notions of privacy and confidentiality. Elsewhere in the world, where a whole family may take part in the patient's narrative, adding to and elaborating on the story, privacy and confidentiality are nearly impossible and may not even be acceptable. Similarly, involuntary treatment like the use of injectable medications without a patient's consent evokes both modern and traditional objections in the West. After all, the body is a fortress, the abode of a rather easily corrupted and influenced soul. Where soul is an adamantine entity, and a body only its transient abode, as in India (Desai 1989), such intrusions may invoke neither the wrath of the patient (when the family may urge the physician to institute the treatment against a patient's protests) nor the specter of the law.

Bell (1969) described another phenomenon in developing countries that is somewhat alien to Western tenets: "the family in the hospital." Serious and not so serious illnesses bring the whole family to the doctor's office or the hospital. Such a rich support system alters the course of illness and facilitates judicious use of that system in the treatment and care of the patient. No psychiatric evaluation can be complete without an investigation of the patient's support system; and, for those reliant on it, any lack or scarcity of it (such as in the case of lone immigrants) may lead to a need for special attention.

Cultural Elements of the Relationship Between Patient and Clinician

Transference is a stereotypical way of relating to others. The transference figures are subject not only to the unconscious attribution of attitudes and beliefs from the earlier developmental phases, but also to attributions and expectations related to one's cultural assumptions—some conscious, some not so conscious. If a person comes from a culture where relationships are hierarchical, it stands to reason that a clinician, a person with authority, will be treated with deference. A patient in this situation may be overcompliant and may have difficulty disagreeing with the therapist. The therapist from a Western society may attempt to promote autonomy, which may be experienced by the patient as distancing at best, rejecting at worst. The patient may feel that his or her need for unequivocal support is misunderstood as an overdependent attitude.

When patient and therapist are of different genders, culturally ingrained assumptions may also pose difficulties. A male therapist's friendly gesture may be threatening to a female patient, and her normal shyness and reticence may be interpreted by a male therapist as resistance or guilt-laden behavior. Female patients may have difficulty speaking freely about sexual concerns or fantasies, behaviors deemed inappropriate in male–female dialogue. In the reverse situation—a female therapist and a male patient—cultures where men are supposed to be in charge and have higher status make patients regard expression of difficulties as a weakness. Intimacy poses a challenge in either of these pairings. Same-sex relationships are less problematic, especially between female clinicians and female patients (Chin et al. 1993). However, between male patients and male clinicians, misunderstanding around sexually tinged material may also arise. What is crucial is that the traditional and common meaning attributed to these behaviors must be recast in the light of cultural differences. Many cultures do not define gender roles as distinctly as do cultures of the West, particularly the United States; thus a male patient's softness may be misunderstood as feminine strivings and homoerotic orientation.

Language difficulties are surmountable in the hands of sensitive clinicians, for words are a critical but not the only means of communication. If such difficulties occur, they may mask deeper psychopathologies, previously unobserved levels of intelligence, or self-underestimation of the ability to express deeply charged emotions or events. Even when a therapist does not understand the patient's first language, it is often useful to have patients express some charged feelings in their first language, capitalizing on the psychological value of sheer verbalization. In psychotic conditions there may also be language regression, and often the language acquired in adulthood may not be easily available to the patient.

In Western cultures, social status has played a rather powerful role in the treatment of psychiatric patients (Comas-Diaz and Jacobsen 1991). This debate has not been resolved, even though a culturally sensitive, well-trained therapist may feel better equipped to deal with the vicissitudes stemming from ethnic and socioeconomic differences (Chin et al. 1993; Comas-Diaz and Griffith 1987). On the other hand, in most non-Western cultures, age is often connected with status. Older clinicians are therefore natural recipients of a patient's regard and admiration. Younger clinicians, on the other hand, especially when treating older patients, have to be sensitive to their initial reticence; patients are not withholding or disparaging but rather need encouragement to unfold themselves.

Overall Cultural Assessment for Diagnosis and Care

The last segment of DSM-IV-TR's outline of cultural formulation allows for a summation of the significant issues discovered in the foregoing cultural areas. Clinicians must marshal their intuitions and inferences and, tentative as they may be, suggest diagnostic modifications based on the available cultural data. Similar symptom complexes may lead to different conclusions about pathogenesis when cultural considerations throw a different light on the patient's story. Cultural considerations are less problematic when reviewing a major mental illness, but even so, care must be exercised. For example, a patient's attribution of power to external influences may be much less malignant than it may appear. Hearing voices and/or seeing visions of dead relatives are common to some cultures. It is always prudent to remember that a statement, in order to be cataloged as a delusion, must not be part of a patient's culturally held beliefs. Character pathology presents the most serious challenge. Values related to authority, autonomy, dependency, deference, sexuality, submissiveness, aggression, passivity, consistency, face saving, and shame are almost always culturally shaped and shared. Lack of attention, or poor attention, to these issues may result in what may be regarded as "snap" diagnosis or misleading and malignant labeling. The price is paid eventually in failed therapeutic encounters and increased patient suffering.

■ Conclusion

Although DSM-IV'S adoption of an outline of a cultural formulation is a fresh start in the appreciation of cultural contributions to diagnosis and treatment, it is far from restoring cultural psychiatry to its rightful place. If "people are what they eat" or "known by the company they keep," or if "they are because they think," why should it be strange, especially to mental health professionals, that they are what they believe? Appendix I of DSM-IV-TR includes a list of several so-called culture-bound syndromes. Perhaps these unique and seemingly exotic syndromes will be better understood with a basic shift in nosological paradigms that a well-used cultural formulation may generate. For the time being, however, the cultural formulation as summarized here can be a rather useful instrument for a comprehensive clinical assessment of any case. In fact, its structure and precepts are a core component in the analysis and discussion of the clinical cases presented in the following chapter.

■ References

Alarcón RD: Culture and psychiatric diagnosis: impact on DSM-IV and ICD-10. Psychiatr Clin North Am 18:449–466, 1995

American Psychiatric Association: Diagnostic and Statistical Manual of Mental Disorders, 4th Edition. Washington, DC, American Psychiatric Association, 1994

American Psychiatric Association: American Psychiatric Association Practice Guidelines for the Treatment of Psychiatric Disorders (Compendium 2000). Washington, DC, American Psychiatric Association, 2000

American Psychiatric Association: Diagnostic and Statistical Manual of Mental Disorders, 4th Edition, Text Revision. Washington, DC, American Psychiatric Association, 2000

Bell J: Family in the Hospital. Chevy Chase, MD, National Institute of Mental Health, 1969

Chin JL, de la Cancela V, Jenkins YM: Diversity in psychotherapy: the politics of race, ethnicity and gender. Westport, CT, Praeger, 1993

Comas-Diaz L, Griffith E (eds): Clinical guidelines in cross-cultural mental health. New York, Wiley, 1987

Comas-Diaz L, Jacobsen FM: Ethnocultural transference and countertransference in the therapeutic dyad. Am J Orthopsychiatry 61:392–402, 1991

Desai P: Health and Medicine in the Hindu Tradition. New York, Crossroads, 1989

Desai P, Coehlo G: Cultural aspects of psychological adaptation, in New Ethnics: The Case of South Asian Indians. Edited by Saran P, James E. New York, Praeger, 1986, pp 136–142

Desai P, Collins A: Selfhood in context: some Indian solutions, in Cultural Transition. Edited by White M, Pollok S. Boston, Routledge and Kegan Paul, 1985, pp 98–106

Durkheim E: Suicide: A Study in Sociology. Glencoe, IL, Free Press, 1951

Erikson E: Childhood and Society. New York, WW Norton, 1950

Erikson E: Identity and the life cycle: selected papers, in Psychological Issues. New York, International Universities Press, 1959, pp 10–150

Fabrega H: Cultural and historical foundations of psychiatric diagnosis, in Culture and Psychiatric Diagnosis: A DSM-IV Perspective. Edited by Mezzich JE, Kleinman A, Fabrega H, et al. Washington, DC, American Psychiatric Press, 1996, pp 3–14

Gedo JE, Goldberg A: Models of the Mind: A Psychoanalytic Theory. Chicago, University of Chicago Press, 1973

Good BJ: Epilogue: knowledge, power and diagnosis, in Culture and Psychiatric Diagnosis. A DSM-IV Perspective. Edited by Mezzich JE, Kleinman A, Fabrega H, et al. Washington, DC, American Psychiatric Press, 1996, pp 347–351

Kakar S: Shamans, Mystics and Doctors. New York, Alfred A. Knopf, 1982

Kleinman A: Depression, Somatization and the New Cross-Cultural Psychiatry. Social Science and Medicine 11:3–10, 1977

Kleinman A: Rethinking Psychiatry. New York, Free Press, 1988

Kleinman A: Writing at the Margins: Discourse Between Anthropology and Medicine. Berkeley, CA, University of California Press, 1996

Lukoff D, Lu FG, Turner R: Cultural considerations in the assessment and treatment of religious and spiritual problems. Psychiatr Clin North Am 18:467–485, 1995

Marriott M: Constructing an Indian ethnosociology, in India through Hindu Categories. Edited by Marriott M. New Delhi, Sage, 1990, pp 38–48

McGoldrick M, Pearce JK, Giodano J (eds): Ethnicity and Family Therapy. New York, Guilford, 1996

Menninger K: A Manual for Psychiatric Case Study. New York, Grune & Stratton, 1962

Mezzich JE: Cultural Formulation and Comprehensive Diagnosis: Clinical and Research Perspectives. Psychiatr Clin North Am 18: 649–657, 1995

Mezzich J, Kleinman A, Fabrega H, et al (eds): Revised Cultural Psychiatry Proposals for DSM-IV (Technical Report). Pittsburgh, PA, NIMH Culture and Diagnosis Group, 1993

Nichter M: Idioms of distress: alternatives in the expression of psychological distress: a case study from South India. Cult Med Psych 5:379–408, 1981

Nurcombe B, Gallagher RM: The clinical process in psychiatry: diagnosis and management planning. Cambridge, England, Cambridge University Press, 1986

Sampson E: The decentralization of identity: toward a revised concept of personal and social order. Am Psychol 40:1203–1211, 1988

Shweder R, Bourne E: Does the concept of the person vary cross-culturally? in Cultural Conceptions of Mental Health and Therapy. Edited by Marsella A, White CO. New York, Reidal Publishing, 1992

4

DSM-IV-TR Cultural Formulation Applied to Six Clinical Cases

■ Drugs Are Shame

This case illustrates the complex interaction of culture and human behavior. Bound to the traditions of the old country, yet American by birth and socialization, this patient (the son of Irish Catholic immigrants) struggles with sexual conflicts, issues of identity shaped by strong religious precepts, and a personality riddled with guilt, shame, and confusion. This creates self-doubt and ultimately leads the patient to depression, heavy drinking, and violent behavior. This case also explores the role of women, family hierarchies, and communication patterns in the household, their influence on the socialization of the child, and their continuity in shaping personality and conflicts in adulthood.

Identifying Data

Mr. A is a 42-year-old, single, college-educated white male. He is a first-generation Irish American, the son of an Irish Catholic immigrant couple.

Reason for Evaluation

Mr. A complained of problems in his sexual relationships and thoughts and behaviors that had disturbed him most of his adult life. He stated that he was "at the end of the rope" and could no longer tolerate his worry and feelings of guilt about his compulsion to masturbate.

History of Present Illness

Although of long duration, Mr. A's problems became particularly trouble-some when several years ago he moved in with a woman friend, with whom he shared intellectual, recreational, and social interests. He reported that he had lost interest in her sexually shortly after their relationship became serious. He became shy and inhibited in her presence and embarrassed to look at her body and to expose his own. He confessed, somewhat reluctantly, that masturbating was preferable to the "real thing," about which he felt intense shame. He enjoyed "girlie magazines," which he would hide. When his girlfriend discovered the magazines, she berated him for his inattention to her and for his "perverse interests." He resented her "putting demands" on him. He withdrew even more and tried, although unsuccessfully, to be more discreet and secretive about his masturbation, but she continued to find his rehidden materials. The scenario of worry, being discovered, and experiencing shame has repeated itself throughout his life.

Immediately prior to his coming to treatment, Mr. A's girlfriend's reactions escalated. She talked of suicide if they split up and felt that she was unable to cope with his preference for girlie magazines and mastur-bation rather than for sexual relations with her. He felt increasingly guilty and became depressed. Despite his efforts, however, he could not control his urges to masturbate. He felt weak and ashamed and believed that he was a "pervert."

Mr. A also expressed concerns about his aversion to marriage, the idea of which created intense anxiety. He felt guilty that he was not "man enough" to give his girlfriend what he felt she deserved, marriage and children. In her presence he felt like a "bad boy," chastised by her at every turn. To distance himself from these concerns, he spent every evening at the bar with his male friends, playing cards and drinking. He attempted to assuage his guilt feelings by attending religious services and by confession. There was no history of homosexuality—feelings, acting out, or relationships.

Past Psychiatric History

There was no previous history of psychiatric treatment.

General Medical History

Mr. A was an inveterate jogger and swimmer but feared the risks associated with his smoking, drinking, and drug use. He had no history of significant medical illnesses and no signs or symptoms of illness at the time of coming for treatment. Liver function tests were negative.

History of Substance Abuse

Mr. A admitted to a serious problem with alcohol, which had begun in college when he was 21 years old. He would drink during lunch breaks and was often tipsy in class. He continued a pattern of heavy drinking and at the time of entering treatment had had a hangover every morning for the previous 5 years. He denied having DTs, hallucinations, or blackouts, and he had never been treated for alcohol dependency. He smoked two packs of cigarettes and drank four to five cups of coffee a day. He admitted to using marijuana on several occasions but denied the use of other illicit drugs.

Developmental History

Mr. A was born in a large Northeastern city, the youngest of five children and the only boy. He remembered being his mother's favorite child and being doted on by his sisters, like their "doll-baby" to dress up and feed. He recalled being dressed in his sister's cast-off clothing and his hair being left to grow to shoulder length during his preschool years.

Mr. A's piously religious mother was described as a "Jekyll and Hyde," who had the habit of turning on him with fury, then expressing remorse afterwards. He defended himself against his mother's unpredictable behavior by using his wit, charm, and humor to ensure her good mood, and he recalled the place where he sat in the kitchen entertaining her with jokes and stories while she worked. He remembered vividly an occasion on which she lashed him with a strap because she thought he was clumsy to have fallen off his bicycle, bruising his knees and head.

Mr. A grew up with a strict Catholic upbringing. He dutifully went to church with his mother every Sunday and observed all holy days in

household rituals. He remembered catechism classes, his first commun-
ion, and the vow he took on his confirmation day not to drink alcohol
until his twenty-first birthday. This pleased his mother, who thought that
if her son kept to "the straight and narrow," he might someday be called
to serve the Church as a priest.

As an adolescent, Mr. A began to understand how difficult the straight
and narrow path was, and he struggled with the issue of sin daily. He
recalls one evening when his sisters had a sleepover with their girlfriends.
The girls practiced ballet exercises in their underclothes in an open room
adjacent to his own. He pretended to be asleep but was watching them,
became aroused, and quietly masturbated beneath the covers. He felt intense guilt and confessed this to the priest the next day. On the way
home after completing the required penance, he thought of yet another
sexual idea and felt an urge to return to confession. His behavior soon
became fanatical, with daily rituals of masturbation followed by confession. Since he could not give up masturbating, he decided that he could
no longer go to church, which created a sense of loss in his life. His mother responded to his not going to church by whipping him, and after that
she never ceased to admonish him.

His father was an alcoholic whose wife resented his drinking. During
Mr. A's boyhood, his father was seldom home in the evenings; he preferred spending his time with male friends at the neighborhood bar. The
father had stopped going to church during his own adolescence, and he
remained silent when his son stopped going to church. The father had
been and continued to be silent about most issues.

Social History

On coming to treatment, Mr. A was living with his girlfriend and had remained scrupulously monogamous in this relationship despite his sexual
preoccupations. He was a professor in a large university, where he teach-
es sociology. The major focus of his research and teaching was deviant
behavior. He continued to drink daily but was able to function relatively
well and to hide his alcoholism and deviant behaviors. So far Mr. A had
not had problems at work or with the law.

Occupational History

After graduation from a Catholic university, Mr. A worked as an under-
cover law enforcement agent. His mission was to observe the activities of
alleged prostitutes and then to arrest them. He was fascinated with his

job, but soon found himself feeling sorry for these women. He befriended one who, for a short time, moved in with him, causing him conflict and guilt. Once again he had to hide his immoral, illegal behavior from authority figures (his job supervisors). He decided to leave this job because he felt guilty that he was being drawn into this "sordid life." He went to graduate school, pursued sociology, and wrote his graduate dissertation on the subject of deviance. His preoccupation in both his personal and professional life has since focused continually on issues of good versus sinful behavior.

Family History

Mr. A's father died several years ago at age 75 of alcoholic cirrhosis. His mother was still living when he came to treatment and had no known medical or psychiatric problems. Two of Mr. A's sisters were single professional women who were dependent on alcohol and drank heavily on a daily basis. His other two sisters— one a married housewife with children, the other a Catholic nun—were without medical or psychiatric problems.

Physical Examination and Review of Systems

Physical examination was essentially unremarkable. He exhibited no tremors and no physical stigmata of drinking or drug use. Review of systems was negative.

Mental Status Examination

Mr. A, a healthy-looking, athletic man of normal stature, was casually but stylishly dressed. He made good eye contact and was very cooperative and articulate. On occasion he joked and made witty, insightful remarks. There was no pressure of speech or abnormal motor behaviors. In a ritualistic manner, he described his worry and concern about repeated episodes: leaving his office—buying girlie magazines—going to his apartment, drinking some beer, and masturbating—hiding the magazines—taking a shower—returning to his office—feeling guilt and self-reproach throughout the day—dreading pressure for intimacy from his girlfriend—and rather than facing her, going to the bar to drink and to feel sorry, then finally going home to face her disdain and criticism of his "perverted" behavior.

He stated, "If I just think of smoking, drinking, or masturbating—it's as if I've actually done it—I'm a lowlife—I might as well sink into it all the way—then I won't stop myself from doing it." There was no evidence of other morbid ideas, worries, or preoccupations, and there were no delusions or hallucinations. He expressed a desire to stop smoking, drinking, and masturbating and a yearning for spiritual development. He feared going to church because of the sin in his life.

Formal mental status, including cognitive functions was normal. His insight was good, but his judgment was impaired, evidenced by his extreme risk-taking behaviors, i.e., heavy drinking and drug use.

DSM-IV-TR Diagnosis

Axis I
1. Alcohol dependence
2. Sexual aversion disorder
3. Dysthymic disorder

Axis II
Personality disorder NOS with narcissistic and obsessive-compulsive traits

Axis III
None

Axis IV
Psychosocial stressors: conjugal discord, severity 3 (moderate) and enduring
Religious problem

Axis V
GAF=75 (current)

Case Summary

Mr. A's history revealed a strong family diathesis for alcohol dependency. His father was alcohol dependent and died of cirrhosis, two older sisters were heavy, daily drinkers, and his mother, although a more moderate drinker, suffered severe mood swings during his early childhood years secondary to her alcohol use. Throughout his adult years, Mr. A had manifested dependency on alcohol, nicotine, and caffeine, which also served to modulate his tension states.

Mr. A experienced feelings of guilt on the one hand, but resentment and rebelliousness on the other, because of ambivalent and, at times, harsh childhood experiences regarding his "sins," now alcohol and sex. He continued to struggle with his perceived badness and that of others, through his research, his professional endeavors, and his search for forgiveness via confession in church, to his mother, and to his girlfriend. He feared chastisement and submissively sought acceptance, approval, and love from authority figures as he had as a boy from his mother.

These unresolved conflicts have caused significant problems in his adult relationships. Despite his desire to be with a woman, he is conflicted about a sexual relationship and deeply afraid of the responsibilities of marriage and children. He retreats regressively to visual images and to masturbating as he did in adolescence while he secretly watched his sisters and their friends dance in their underwear. His girlfriend's admonishments about his "perverse behavior" reinforces his belief that he is bad and reinforces his morbid, recurrent behavioral cycles: sin-guilt-shame-remorse.

Cultural Formulation

Cultural Identity of the Individual

Mr. A's cultural identity is that of an Irish Catholic American. Both of his parents were born in Ireland, moved with their parents to the United States as children, and were raised in a predominantly working-class, Irish American neighborhood. Mr. A had a strongly religious upbringing, attending Catholic schools and catechism classes, and he even felt drawn to the priesthood until his disaffection.

Cultural Explanations of the Individual's Illness

The degree to which Mr. A's behavior would be considered normal rather than pathological might be strongly influenced by the cultural context, as related to his ethnicity, religion, and gender. His drinking habits were not considered unusual by the male friends with whom he drank. Similarly, one might expect such a pious Catholic to struggle with the rightness or wrongness of his sexual desires.

Mr. A however, felt disturbed enough by his behaviors to seek treatment. He recognized the potential medical problems secondary to his excessive use of alcohol and was aware of his father's death due to the complications of alcoholism. His problem drinking and sexual behaviors were known to his girlfriend, who considered them disturbed and perverted, and these behaviors have seriously interfered with his interpersonal relationships and functioning.

Cultural Factors Related to Psychosocial Environment and
Levels of Functioning

Mr. A was a sensitive and intellectual boy, small in stature, who was raised in a household of females. The traditions of Irish songs and music, some Gaelic language, attendance at a predominantly Irish Catholic church, and celebrating St. Patrick's Day were cherished parts of his early childhood experience. He grew up in a poor, tough, Irish neighborhood where only the rowdy male who was able to fight and/or who was member of ganglike groups was able to sustain his sense of manhood. Mr. A was not much of a street fighter, and he therefore derived his social reputation and self-esteem from his quick wit, facile use of language, humor, and charm. Although he was able to talk his way out of the most aggressively threatening situations and loved argumentative debate with his male friends at the neighborhood Irish bar, he found it difficult to hold his own with women. His perception of women (like his perception of his mother) was that "they lose their tempers and all reason takes leave."

As a boy in a household of sisters and their girlfriends (parading in their underwear, as he vividly recalled on one occasion), Mr. A found himself sexually overstimulated, which caused him to feel wicked and sinful. In the context of his Roman Catholic upbringing, such sexual feelings were taboo and dangerous. Fearing the power of his dominating, piously religious mother, and left out of the male world of his father, he became increasingly anxious and conflicted about his budding sexual desires. His compulsive masturbation—which became his way of discharging his sexual tensions, as well as a means of assuring himself of the integrity of his penis (in context of his castration anxiety)—left him feeling ashamed, guilty, remorseful, and in need of chastisement. He defended against these feelings and the associated guilt through "undoing": confessing his sins to make the desires go away and to be relieved of the shame and guilt he felt. This became the model for his adult neurotic problems: sin-guilt-shame-remorse.

Drinking and the neighborhood bar became for Mr. A a method for tension regulation, a forum for masculine solidarity, a refuge from female dominance, and a source for calm and nurturance (ironically, with maternal developmental origins) in the form of the intoxicating beer. Mr. A drinks to get a "buzz" that dulls the pain of his guilt, as well as his sexual desires, and solicits chastisement from his girlfriend. Thus in a rebellious manner he resorts to private masturbation and activates the cycle of sin-guilt-shame-confession.

Cultural Elements of the Relationship Between the
Individual and the Clinician

Mr. A frequently used the phrase, "I must confess...." in an offhand, col-loquial manner in therapy to introduce a litany of what he considered bad behaviors. Exploration of this casual use of an idiom in the transference helped him gain insight into the influences of his Catholic upbringing, his conflicts, his unresolved guilt, and the ways in which these issues contin-ue to be acted out in his current functioning and in his relationships.

Overall Cultural Assessment for Diagnosis and Care

Mr. A's therapy included exploration and understanding of a number of cultural factors inherent in his Irish Catholic upbringing. In this case the specific ethnic factors included

1. Values and attitudes about sex and masturbation in Irish Catholic so-ciety
2. The role of the woman in the household and in the socialization of the child
3. The role of the Church in the socialization of the child
4. Corporal punishment in the household and in parochial schools
5. The role of the eldest and youngest son in the family household
6. The nature of male-male and male-female relationships in Irish Cath-olic society
7. Attitudes and values associated with bars and alcohol use
8. Self-isolation and secrecy versus self-disclosure and confession
9. Therapeutic issues involving transference in an Irish Catholic patient
10. Irish Catholic responses to the structure of Alcoholics Anonymous (AA)
11. The spiritual resolution of internal conflicts

Clinical Course

Mr. A willingly entered an alcohol and drug detoxification and rehabili-tation program. Initially he felt uncomfortable and more guilty in reaction to the religious references in his 12-step program, but he actively partic-ipated in the program. After becoming sober he was able to benefit from expressive psychoanalytic psychotherapy. With sobriety there was an intensification of persistent feelings of low self-esteem, depression, and compulsive behaviors, for which he was treated additionally with clomipramine 25 mg qid.

During the course of psychotherapy Mr. A revealed his fascination and curiosity during his childhood about the difference between his genitals and his sister's and mother's. He remembered that when his sisters would dress him up as a girl, he wondered whether his penis had brought him their attentions. He did not want to show his penis to them, but wanted to "look at the place between their legs" where his penis would be put, which made him feel very guilty. In the absence of his father he had no model for identification and no means to understand these feelings, and he felt overwhelmed and "unmanly." He wondered whether his mother had been so charmed by him sometimes but rageful at other times because she somehow knew of his sinful thoughts. He feared that his thoughts would be discovered and that he would be punished. To protect himself from these females and the "sinful" feelings they stirred in him, he distanced himself from intimacy with his sisters and mother and forged an identification with his father as he sought solace in the neighborhood bar with his male drinking buddies.

This cycle repeated itself in Mr. A's intimate relationships with women. He felt inferior and frightened by women's advances, demands, and their sexuality—which he felt he could never satisfy and which generated castration anxiety in him. He masturbated as a substitute and to assure protection and integrity of his penis, he felt guilty about his sinful behavior, and he sought forgiveness through confession and being chastised.

Mr. A's ambivalence toward the Church continued, as did his ambivalence toward women (he shied away from personal contact with them in daily life). His continuing need to confess his sins, displaced onto his girlfriend, soon emerged within his treatment and in his AA meetings. As he began to feel identified the therapist (the male authority figure) in the treatment, he began to attend AA meetings every evening instead of going to the bar. Through AA he was reintroduced to spirituality and began to feel more comfortable again with prayer and with his relationship to the God of his Irish Catholic tradition. As he found sobriety, his sense of being a reprobate sinner subsided. He similarly used therapy as a confessional to contain his castration anxiety and to seek absolution and forgiveness from the therapist for his sinful behavior. Interpretation of the transference and reconstruction of the origins of his behavior allowed him to gain insight into his conflicts, his castration anxiety (the sin-guilt-remorse cycle), and his drinking for comfort and self-nurturing.

Mr. A continued to think of marriage and fatherhood as incompatible with what he admitted were his and his mother's earliest, fondest ambitions for him: to become a priest. He had ruled out such an option for himself in youth because of his belief that he was an uncontrollable sinner who could never be accepted by the Church. The pros and cons of such vocational issues became important topics in his psychotherapy. Many psychiatrists might view the choice to enter religious life by this patient as a reflection of unresolved conflicts about intimacy and sexuality (the solution that his mother would have advocated) that would leave his sexuality unfulfilled. On the other hand, it seemed possible that the spiritual solution proposed by entering a religious life and celibacy reflected a cultural belief about what constitutes a fulfilling life. As it should be with every case, this choice was one that only the patient could make, and so he did.

Mr. A began to attend Mass on Sundays, then each morning before work, and he soon felt a sense of belonging there and developed closer, spiritual friendships with several of the priests. Finally, during a week-long religious retreat, he felt called by God to the religious life. He returned home and discussed the matter with his girlfriend, who was well aware of the transformation that had been occurring in Mr. A's life. With some ambivalence, they both decided that living together should not continue. Mr. A's rapprochement with his parental imagoes through the transference in psychotherapy paralleled his rapprochement with the Church fathers (and mothers). He accepted the security of the Church's embrace and moved from boyhood reactions and identifications into an honorable role for an adult Catholic male—that of celibate religious man. He felt at peace with this decision and, for the first time, had ambitions that were free of conflict and guilt.

With the resolution of his conflicts, Mr. A's symptoms subsided, and medications were discontinued without the return of symptoms. He continued in psychotherapy once a week until his entrance into the seminary. He continues his commitment to and involvement in Alcoholics Anonymous.

Discussion

This case illustrates the important role of cultural factors in shaping both normal and pathological behaviors. The profound impact of the Catholic religion on the Irish person, whether church-attending or not, is often inadvertently overlooked, since it is for the most part regarded as a subject beyond the boundaries of the usual psychiatric treatment considerations.

This patient's sexual guilt, which had origins in his early development but was strongly influenced by his Irish Catholic upbringing, interfered with his intimate relationships with women, from whom he distanced himself emotionally, as he similarly created distance from the Catholic Church and God. He became narcissistically invested in himself, developed his mind and wit, paid attention to his appearance, and was admired and found to be amusing by others. He also turned to himself for gratification, stimulated by clandestine glimpses of women through the peepholes in his childhood bedroom and those offered by the photos in girlie magazines and pornographic videos. Substances (alcohol, drugs, caffeine, nicotine) were used for the autoerotic pleasure they induced as well as for the protection and comfort they provided him regarding his castration anxiety. While protecting him from his conflict and anxiety, this defensive posture, as influenced by culture, at the same time, perpetuated a sin-guilt-shame-remorse cycle. His conflicts and the associated defensive patterns revealed a complex interface between his oedipal guilt and culturally derived attitudes and values regarding the nature of women and sexuality, and men and alcohol, in Irish Catholic society.

Religion, sexuality, and alcohol have been interconnected subjects of conflict and topics of debate within Irish culture for centuries. Fundamental to this debate has been the political and economic disempowerment of Irish men, which has contributed to problems in establishing self-esteem and independence from their families of origin (Scheper-Hughes 1979). Sons were duty bound to help eke out a living from the family's marginally productive farm; courtship and sexual activity were usually postponed, and only later in life were men free to marry. These values were reinforced by the Catholic Church. The Church also provided honorable roles and a way out of poverty for both males and females in Irish society through entering religious life. In addition, the Church has been a major influence on values and family life in traditional Ireland. Mothers have commonly encouraged their younger children to become nuns and priests, vocations conveying dignity and pride for the family and within the community.

The traditional Irish household is predominantly mother centered. Mothers often become devoted to a particular son or daughter and vow to raise them to be better than their father. Warnes (1979) reported that there are "a striking number of virgin bachelors over forty" who live with their mothers. From the family's perspective, the father is somewhat inaccessible spending his social time in the pub, which has served as a traditional locale for a home-away-from-home for adult males and has contributed to male camaraderie and solidarity, separating them from the women and children at home. This segregation of men from women in daily life contributes to and is a reflection of sexual repression in Irish society. The Catholic Church condemns all forms of sexuality outside formal marriage. These prohibitions reinforce social incentives to avoid sex. Irish men who drink often say that they need the disinhibition of alcohol because of guilt about sexuality (Teahan 1988).

Despite the camaraderie between males at the pub and the expectation that social networks will be reinforced by hosting with drinks, ambivalence runs deep regarding Irish attitudes toward alcohol. Vaillant (1983) commented that the Irish tend to regard drinking alcohol in terms of moral opposites: good or evil, complete abstinence or drunkenness. As early as 1738, Dr. Samuel Madden, a founder of the Royal Dublin Society, called for laws to "force people to sobriety that they may...feed their families." The first "Anti-spirits" Society was founded in the early 1830s in New Ross County, and the first Alcoholics Anonymous (AA) in Europe was founded in Dublin in 1946 (Walsh 1987). From 1960 onward, 12%–13% of personal expenditure in Ireland went to alcohol—the highest percentage in Europe. O'Conner (1978) surveyed one county in Ireland and found that 24% of all adult males were "heavy drinkers." On the other hand, Walsh (1987) observed that there are actually proportionally fewer drinkers in Ireland than in England and Wales. There is some suggestion that the Irish who drink may drink more and may have more problems. O'Conner (1978) found that, although there are a large number of alcoholics in Ireland, there are also a great number of abstainers. It is a common Church practice for many adolescents to pledge abstinence from alcohol until age 21, as was the case with Mr. A.

The ambivalence with which Irish regard the use of alcohol is portrayed in attitudes within the Church itself. Bales (1962) pointed out that in the Catholic Mass it is only the priest who partakes of the wine. In this act, it is only the priest who thereby comes into contact with the sacred. Here the use of alcohol in religious ritual is epitomized, providing the paradigm for its use on the less formalized but numerous festive and saints' days in the annual calendar. Although the Catholic Church sanctions the use of alcohol for priests in religious contexts, abstinence from alcohol during Lent and until age 21 is considered an act of self-discipline that cleanses the desires of the body for redemption of the soul. Similar values are held regarding abstinence from food and sex.

Among the Irish, drinking alcohol is not associated with ideas about enhancement of courting or sexual performance, as it is with many adolescents and adults in greater United States society (Christiansen and Walsh 1987). On the contrary, Arensberg (1937) pointed out that in Ireland it was often the teetotaler who was suspected of staying sober enough to prowl around the streets getting girls into trouble! Such ideas were reinforced by the observations that the teetotalers were often lone young men, not socially accepted by the "boys" of their own age and class who frequented the pubs. According to Teahan (1988), male solidarity and identification with a clan of males takes place in the pubs over drinks and convivial conversation about politics, sports, and religion, but rarely about sex and women. Masculine prowess was also expressed more aggressively in taunts and fights with rival groups of "boys." Maintaining dominance and prestige required clever rhetoric and physical strength and skill, attributes valued and pursued by Irish men. Teahan points out that the loss of physical strength and ability is a predominant concern among Irish males who drink and has been found to be useful clinically as a motivator for treatment.

Studies have found that the most feared consequence of heavy drinking among the Irish is not physical deterioration, but spiritual: it is feared that drinking will create feelings of depression, shame, and guilt (Teahan 1988). Greeley et al. (1980) and O'Hanlon (1975) commented on the guilt, anxiety, and low self-esteem found among Irish males. A recent study has found that 20% of Irish alcoholics, compared to only 5% of Canadian alcoholics, rate achieving a "sense of detachment" as their highest perceived consequence of drinking (Teahan 1988). The Irish group of heavy drinkers may thereby achieve respite from their guilt but, in doing so, actually perpetuate the self-defeating cycle of guilty behavior that was shown in Mr. A.

Warnes (1979) discussed how this struggle with sin and guilt is frequently reenacted in the treatment situation, where the male Irish patient promises over and over again to try to control his behavior. Warnes believes that this attitude is related to overcompliance but unconscious provocation, originally directed to the mother. In an interpersonal style that Warnes terms "masochistic exhibitionism," those afflicted make every effort to reveal rather than conceal their shortcomings in order to demonstrate how cruel the mother of their childhood was. Because of this dynamic, he speculates that the healing power of Catholic confession may be as effective in some such instances as treatment offered by psychiatrists. In a similar way, as illustrated in this case, as a result of strong cultural influences, the ultimate resolution for internal conflicts may be a spiritual one based on the patient's final life choices.

■ References

Arensberg C: The Irish Countryman. New York, Macmillan, 1937

Bales RF: Attitudes towards drinking in the Irish culture, in Society, Culture and Drinking Patterns. Edited by Pittman DJ, Synder CR. New York, Wiley, 1962, pp 91–112

Christiansen B, Walsh J: Cross-cultural comparisons of Irish and American adolescent drinking: practices and beliefs. J Stud Alcohol 48:558–562, 1987

Greeley A, McCready W, Theisen G: Ethnic Drinking Subcultures. Brooklyn, NY, JF Bergian, 1980

O'Conner J: The Young Drinkers: A Cross-National Study of Social and Cultural Influences. London, Tavistock Publishing, 1978

O'Hanlon T: The Irish. New York, Harper & Row, 1975

Scheper-Hughes N: Saints, Scholars and Schizophrenics: Mental Illness in Rural Ireland. Berkeley, CA, University of California Press, 1979

Teahan J: Alcohol Expectancies of Irish and Canadian Alcoholics. International Journal of the Addictions 23:1057–1070, 1988

Vaillant G: The Natural History of Alcoholism. Cambridge, MA, Harvard University Press, 1983

Walsh D: Alcohol and Ireland. British Journal of Addiction 52:118–120, 1987

Warnes H: Cultural Factors in Irish Psychiatry. Psychiatric Journal of the University of Ottawa 4:329–335, 1979

■ A Pakistani Family Affair

A relatively recent phenomenon of migration is that people go abroad for what is intended to be a time-limited period, primarily for advanced education and specialized work experience, but then decide to remain as immigrants. The differences in cultural traditions between the immigrants and the society of their new country may create conflicts for the individual and/or family and lead to significant emotional stress. These issues are illustrated in this case of a Pakistani Muslim family who came to the United States with the intention of returning home when the patient's husband had completed residency training in surgery. The resultant acculturative stress and its impact on the family members is discussed in the theoretical context of the psychosocial outcome of acculturation.

Identifying Data

Ms. B is a 46-year-old woman, married and mother of four children. She was born in a large city in Pakistan and trained there as a nurse. Shortly after she graduated, she married a recent medical graduate she had met while working at the same hospital. One month later the couple migrated to the United States, where they had been living for more than 20 years at the time the patient came for treatment.

Reason for Evaluation

Ms. B's relationship with her husband, Dr. B, had been deteriorating for many months. A recent family visit to Pakistan had exacerbated strains between her and her in-laws. She had been feeling humiliated, angry, and suspicious of her husband's motives and behavior. She felt overwhelmed, unable to cope, hopeless, and resentful, to the point that she was having thoughts of giving up and fears of hurting herself or one of the children. She reluctantly agreed to a psychiatric consultation.

History of Present Illness

Ms. B's relationship with her husband, a successful surgeon, had been strained for many years. With the move to the United States, she felt isolated and cut off from family and friends. She endured difficult circumstances, and she made many sacrifices during his residency training, including what could have been a promising career for herself in nursing. He ignored and ridiculed her when she expressed concerns about his drinking and his being overly friendly with other women. Similarly, whenever she attempted to discuss her feelings about his sister, with whom she had a difficult relationship, or whenever there was a disagreement between her and her sister-in-law, he would disregard her position and side with his sister. She felt humiliated, angry, and helpless at those times.

In addition to the ongoing strain in her marriage, for several months prior to admission Ms. B had been worried about her 20-year-old daughter, the oldest child. Her daughter was doing poorly academically, had difficulties making friends, and felt isolated and generally unhappy at college. Although she had never been on her own, the daughter had decided to move to a city far from home and known for its high rate of violent crime. Preoccupied with her daughter's predicament, Ms. B became anxious, restless, irritable, distracted, and unable to sleep. Her mood was depressed and labile, with frequent crying spells. She complained of poor appetite, fatigue, and a loss of interest in household activities. She felt too tired to keep up her usual activities at the Muslim Community Center, which had been a major social outlet for her. She blamed her husband for their daughter's problems, and communication between her and her husband deteriorated.

Two months prior to admission Ms. B and her family returned from a 6-week visit to Pakistan. During this visit the children objected to the restrictions placed on their behavior in Pakistan, causing arguments between them and their grandmother and subsequent disputes between the patient and her husband. As usual, her husband sided with his family, criticizing Ms. B for her lack of control over the children. Ms. B had returned from that visit feeling demoralized, angry, and humiliated.

Several weeks prior to admission Ms. B became more agitated and labile. She withdrew to her room, argued frequently with her husband, and was impatient and intolerant with the children. She was convinced that her husband was listening in on her phone conversations with her sister, taping them, and planning to use them against her. She thought that her husband's sister had put an evil spell on her to cause misfortune to befall their older daughter, and she thought that worse things would surely happen. She felt like giving up and stabbing herself at one moment and lashing out at her husband or children the next moment.

Although the patient had received treatment previously (see "Past Psychiatric History" below) she had not seen a psychiatrist nor been taking medication for 6 months prior to admission.

Past Psychiatric History

Ms. B had felt the strain in her marital relationship for nearly 10 years and had felt sad, lonely, isolated, and suspicious of her husband's behavior. Neither she nor her husband, however, regarded her concerns or behavior as symptomatic of any psychiatric problem. When she became more persistently angry and accusatory about his behavior, Dr. B prevailed on a fellow Pakistani, a medical school classmate who had subsequently trained in psychiatry in the United States, to provide an informal consultation for Ms. B at the psychiatrist's home, as part of a social visit. Ms. B was very reluctant to do this because the two couples were friends and she felt that her husband wanted this consultation for his benefit rather than hers. Despite her reservations, the consultation took place. Because of concerns about the stigma that would be associated with a psychiatric diagnosis, it was agreed that any medication prescribed would be monitored by both the patient's husband and the psychiatrist.

Ms. B was started on trifluoperazine, 5–10 mg/day. She disliked the side effects that she experienced from the medication, including dry mouth, constipation, tremor, blurred vision, fatigue, and weight gain; she therefore wanted to decrease the dosage and ultimately stopped taking it after 6 months. Her husband adamantly disagreed with her decision, and he had been advised by the psychiatrist friend to urge her to resume taking it and even to increase the dose when she became more irritable, angry, and frustrated with him. The couple struggled constantly over the issue of the medication, and this unstructured and unsupervised treatment went on for over 5 years. The patient became increasingly more convinced that she should not accept treatment from someone who represented her husband's interests more than her own.

Two years prior to this admission, Ms. B had agreed to consult with a psychiatrist who was neither Pakistani nor previously known to her nor her husband and who practiced at the academic center in the city in which they lived. She was placed on haloperidol, developed akathisia, and was changed to perphenazine, 8 mg/day. She took the medication only intermittently over a 2-year period because she was unconvinced that she needed it and because she experienced side effects.

Medical History and Physical Examination

Ms. B had been in good physical health all of her life. She complained of being overweight and unable to lose weight but had no physical symptoms. She was not taking medication for any medical disorder at the time of her admission, nor had she in years past. She had no history of drug allergies.

History of Substance Abuse

Ms. B was a strictly observant Muslim and had never used alcohol or street drugs.

Psychosocial/Developmental History

Ms. B was born into a financially secure, socially prominent family in Pakistan, the second of three girls. Her family was deeply affected by the factionalism, civic turmoil, and violence that followed Indian and Pakistani independence. During this time thousands of families fled for their lives and parents became separated from their children. Ms. B ended up in a massive camp for displaced persons in her preteen years until her parents were able to find her more than 6 months later. After this experience she felt insecure and anxious for many months and vulnerable in her relationships with family and friends.

Ms. B attended elite private schools and was an accomplished student. After high school graduation she entered nursing training, performed well, and had planned to go to graduate school. Instead, her marriage was arranged in the traditional Muslim manner by her family. Her husband-to-be was a promising young student from a rural community, the only son and the middle of three children. The couple met while working at the same hospital and were married when Dr. B graduated. Soon thereafter they migrated to the United States so that he could begin residency training in surgery. They had planned to stay only as long as was necessary for Dr. B to complete his training in surgery, then return to Pakistan. His plan was to become a surgeon at the university hospital where they had both trained and later to establish a private surgical clinic. Realizing that his career opportunities would be much more rewarding and easier to develop in the United States, they decided to stay for at least 5 more years to accumulate enough money to build a house and establish a private surgical clinic in Pakistan before returning there to live. The couple had four children—two girls, followed by two boys, all 1–2 years apart. They planned to make regular visits and to design a home in Pakistan to accommodate Dr. B's mother and older sister, as well as their own growing family.

Over time the couple's plans were altered. Ms. B became increasingly unhappy about the expectations that her husband and his family had about how she should conduct herself in Pakistan. She was expected to defer at all times to the wishes of her mother-in-law, and she was not being permitted to maintain close ties with her own family and friends. She felt that her mother-in-law envied Ms. B's higher social class and disapproved of her and her family's more liberal views, particularly about advanced education and careers for women. As the children grew into teenagers, they increasingly objected to spending their vacations in Pakistan. The children, who regarded themselves as Americans and not accustomed to Pakistani ways of life, openly objected to being expected to behave in the traditional ways demanded by their grandmother and supported by their father.

The family's annual visits to Pakistan became increasingly more contentious. Ms. B was angry and resentful that her husband always took the side of his mother and sister against her and their children and unhappy about the large amount of money he was investing in the house and his clinic in Pakistan. After supporting the immigration of his younger sister and her family to the United States, Dr. B spent large sums of money setting up a business for his sister's husband, but he had done little to assist Ms. B's sister and brother-in-law, whom he had brought to the United States 2 years earlier. Ms. B's relationship with her sister-in-law and with Dr. B deteriorated. She felt that her sister-in-law manipulated Dr. B to provide more for her than he should and that he always disregarded Ms. B's concerns and sided with his sister. The idea of sharing a house with her husband's mother and older sister in Pakistan grew increasingly less appealing to her.

Dr. B also became disillusioned about the plans to return to Pakistan as he began to realize how difficult it would be to find the technical resources necessary to maintain the standards of professional practice he had become accustomed to in the United States Additionally, the aspirations he had for his children seemed increasingly less realistic. He had hoped that his daughters would complete their education in the United States; through their contacts at the Muslim Community Center, meet suitable young men with whom marriages could be arranged; and return to Pakistan to live. He had hoped that at least one of his sons would become a doctor and eventually take over his practice. The children, however, did not seem interested in these directions.

These social and family factors had caused increasing strain on the marital relationship of the Bs throughout the more than 20 years of their marriage. The impact on Ms. B was a progressive deterioration in her self-esteem, increasing mistrust of her husband, and resentment of her mother-in-law and sister-in-law. She felt rejected, powerless, and helpless. She was angry with her husband and intensely worried about her children's future.

Occupational History

Ms. B had abandoned her plans to become a nurse following her marriage and migration to the United States. She did not work on a permanent basis in the United States and soon had four children to take care of. She worked occasionally as a receptionist at her husband's medical office and did volunteer work in Muslim organizations throughout the years.

Family History

Although Ms. B reported no family history of psychiatric illness, it was reported by her husband that her mother was "emotionally unstable" and had had at least one episode of an acute mental illness. It was not known whether Ms. B's mother had ever seen a psychiatrist or taken psychotropic medications. There is no known psychiatric illness in any other member of her extended family.

Physical Examination

Physical examination and routine laboratory tests on admission were within normal limits.

Mental Status Examination

Although initially guarded, defensive, and difficult to establish rapport with, as the interview progressed Ms. B became more relaxed, able to maintain contact, and cooperative in giving information. She was a mildly obese woman, had no mannerisms, and was striking in her appearance. She wore a colorful silk sari, hair carefully braided, a diamond stud in her nose, gold bracelets on both wrists, and rings on several fingers of both hands. She was oriented to person, place, and time. She appeared sad, tearful, and irritable. Her mood ranged from depressed to agitated and angry but was congruent with thought content. Memory for recent and remote events was intact.

Although fluent in English, Ms. B spoke with a strong accent (her primary language was Urdu) with rapid, pressured speech, and she was difficult to comprehend. There was no evidence of visual or auditory hallucinations. There were ideas of reference and paranoid, delusional ideations. She was convinced that her husband had been listening in on her telephone conversations with her sister and was taping those calls to use against her. She felt that her sisters-in-law were envious of her and her family, had cast an evil spell on the family, and were responsible for the problems that Ms. B's older daughter had been experiencing in recent months. She was convinced that more misfortune would befall her, her children, and/or her husband.

Ms. B felt that she was barely coping; she was worried and worn out and just wanted to give up. She felt helpless, hopeless, powerless, and inadequate. She denied any previous suicidal attempts, but she did admit that she felt like stabbing herself or lashing out at her children and husband. She evidenced some limited insight. She recognized the stress within the family and understood her frustrations and their impact on her sense of adequacy and self-esteem. She was particularly concerned that whenever she disagreed with her husband, he would use her admission to the hospital to label her as "crazy" and to pressure her once again to take drugs she felt were harmful to her.

Functional Assessment

Ms. B had experienced a decrease in the quality of her everyday activities.

Diagnostic Tests

Routine blood work revealed no abnormalities. No additional psychological tests were administered.

DSM-IV-TR Diagnosis

Axis I

Major depressive disorder, recurrent; moderate severity, with psychotic features
Acculturation problem

Axis II

Personality disorder NOS (with borderline and dependent personality traits)

Axis III

None

Axis IV

Marital strain; moderate severity, chronic
Family turmoil; moderate severity, chronic
Acculturative stress, moderate to severe, chronic

Axis V

GAF prior to admission=40
Highest GAF in year following admission=70
Highest GAF in final year of outpatient treatment=90

Case Summary and Differential Diagnosis

Ms. B had begun to experience mood instability during the first years of living in the United States. She felt sad, lonely, and socially isolated, would distance herself emotionally from her husband, and seemed to find little pleasure in her day-to-day activities. She felt unhappy and frustrated in her marriage, and undermined by her husband and in-laws, and she was mistrustful of her husband's intentions and behavior. Her depressive episodes were precipitated by transition to a new culture, by marital and family stress, and by the commonly encountered conflicts of women who marry into and are thereafter bound by the behavioral constrictions imposed by the husband's family. This applied especially to the dictates of the cultural traditions of the husband's mother, whose opinions were expected to govern the behavior of her son's wife and subsequently the next generation. Ms. B's bouts of depression were chronic and recurrent.

Ms. B expressed her distress in terms of what was for her the culturally appropriate belief in malign magic: that her sister-in-law was somehow exerting an evil influence over her and her family that would inevitably bring grave misfortune to them. She accused her husband of violating the code of behavior required of their Muslim religious observance—by drinking alcohol and by displaying overly friendly behavior with (American) women who were not members of his extended family. In the absence of objective verification of the charges about her husband and sister, and in a cultural context, whether her thoughts were delusional might be debatable. (Cultural dynamics will be discussed further in "Cultural Formulation" below.)

During the 6 months prior to admission, the patient's condition deteriorated more substantially, with major depressive symptomatology (agitated depression), vegetative symptoms, mood-congruent ideas of reference, and paranoid delusional ideations. She became impulsive and expressed desires to harm herself or a family member. Her symptoms did meet criteria for a major depressive disorder, with thoughts and behavior that appeared to be of paranoid delusional proportions. However, as the acuity of Ms. B's symptoms diminished, her explanatory framework for her distress shifted more to culturally syntonic ideas about Fate and Divine Will—beliefs widely accepted within the Muslim community in the United States as well as in Pakistan.

Cultural Formulation

Cultural Identity of the Individual

Ms. B was very clear in her cultural identity as an upper-middle-class, urban, educated Pakistani Muslim woman. She usually wore and felt more comfortable in her traditional Pakistani-style clothes, jewelry, and hairstyle. In the United States, her cultural reference groups were primarily other Pakistanis of similar background and other Muslims. Her contact with the wider community was limited primarily to personnel at her children's schools and at the stores where she shopped.

Although Ms. B's comprehension of English was very good, her fluency in spoken English was limited by her rapid speech and strong accent. She had a "Pakistani" rather than an American vocal cadence that made it difficult to understand her. Her primary language was Urdu, which she spoke with her husband, her sister and sister-in-law, and their families. With Pakistani friends, Ms. B spoke a combination of Urdu and English. With her children she spoke mainly Urdu, even when the children responded in English and objected to conversing in Urdu. Because of her limited contact with the community at large, Ms. B never felt confident speaking English and tended to withdraw from social interactions that required greater fluency than she thought she had. As a result, her spoken English changed little during the more than two decades she lived in the United States,

Both Ms. B and her husband had strong ties to their families of origin. Their behavioral norms were those of their Pakistani upbringing, focused on strict adherence to Muslim tradition, deference to parental expectations, and close, supportive relationships with family. A substantial number of Pakistanis lived in the area where the family lived, and Dr. B had a prominent role in the Muslim Community Center, which the couple helped to establish and actively supported. They were involved in numerous social events at the Center and Ms. B often spent considerable time preparing food and helping to organize various events. The couple hoped that their children's social lives would also revolve around the Center so that they would meet and ultimately marry the children of other Pakistani Muslims. The husband was very devout in his adherence to the daily prayer schedule and to ritual behaviors expected of him. He urged Ms. B to be equally observant, but she never shared his degree of commitment, which was a great disappointment to him.

Dr. B is an ardent golfer who plays regularly on weekends and during an annual 2-week spring vacation. He did not involve his wife in any of the activities or friendships connected with his golfing, nor did he encourage her to become involved in any social activities associated with his professional life at the hospital or with his colleagues and their families. Ms. B had no close friends, but with the addition of the numerous school-related activities in which the children were involved, she felt that she had a great deal to handle in her day-to-day life. She regretted, however, her lack of social contacts and involvement in the wider community, was clear that she did not want to return to Pakistan to live, and yearned to take some courses at the regional community college to increase her fluency in English and expand her social contacts.

Cultural Explanations of the Individual's Illness

Ms. B's explanation of her illness was that of malign magic: an evil spell had been placed on her by her sister-in-law. Ms. B was the innocent victim of envious and resentful perpetrators. She felt that her in-laws envied her because of the upper-middle-class, socially prominent status of her family and because of her family's more liberal views about the education and professional advancement of women. These explanations are consistent with the cultural beliefs of the community in which she grew up. Although Ms. B generally denied beliefs in such malign magic, she reverted (as is usually the case) to these cultural beliefs at times of acute stress and emotional vulnerability. With her recovery, these convictions faded into the background of her consciousness and preoccupation. They changed from ego-syntonic beliefs, in the context of her acute distress, to ego-dystonic beliefs, ambivalently held, at other times. When her self-esteem and coping ability were intact, she would deny any belief in malign magic.

The family deferred seeking formal treatment for Ms. B until the severity of her illness could no longer be kept hidden. As a matter of fact, they had attempted to keep it secret by getting a social friend to informally evaluate and treat her through her husband. This is consistent with her culture, in which mental illness is viewed as a great misfortune for the sufferer and the entire family. The knowledge in the community that a given family has a mentally ill member diminishes the marriage prospects of all family members.

Cultural Factors Related to Psychosocial Environment and Levels of Functioning

Ms. B struggled to cope with the inherent conflict between trying to meet the expectations of a traditional Pakistani Muslim family-centered life while simultaneously adapting to living in a country whose customs were unfamiliar and in some respects strange and frightening. During the early years of her marriage, while her husband was consumed with the expectations of his surgical residency training, she had no family or friends to help in her transition and adaptation to life in the United States. This stressful experience became more intense with the birth of their first two children during those years. Burdened by the child care needs of her family and without the emotional and material support she would have had at home in Pakistan, she had a sense of isolation and overwhelming responsibility.

Ms. B's lack of experience in living away from home before marriage, her limited verbal fluency in English, and the family's limited financial resources during Dr. B's residency training contributed to the degree of acculturative stress. It was in the context of this stress that Ms. B felt most isolated, vulnerable, and lonely. With her husband's attentions turned elsewhere, she accused him of betraying her and his own religious principles by drinking and being excessively familiar with other women.

Ms. B had sacrificed home, family, friends, and her career to support her husband's training. While she struggled with taking care of home and family in this new environment, he was unrestricted in his activities outside the home, established a network of friends through his professional life, and was able to make a much more successful integration within the wider community. In later years she was also blamed and held responsible for the children's problems and behavior as they struggled to cope with the conflicts between the traditions of their family and the broader American culture. She was angry, envious, and resentful.

The longer Ms. B lived in the United States, the more difficult and intolerable it became for her to conform to the traditional Pakistani role expectations of a daughter-in law. She was expected to defer to her mother-in-law's opinions concerning proper social behavior for herself and her children and to accept the sanctity and primacy of her husband's obligations to provide for the needs of his family of origin, who had contributed materially to his education. The wife's place in the status hierarchy of her husband's family was age related, and she was also expected to defer to other married women in the family who were older than she. The conflict at first with the mother-in-law and later with the sister-in-law grew steadily over the years. It reached such proportions that Ms. B became less interested in carrying out the original plan to move back to Pakistan in a house designed to also accommodate her husband's mother and sister. For similar reasons, in later years she refused her husband's wishes to bring his mother, who had had a stroke, to live with them in the United States, where Ms. B would be expected to care for her mother-in-law as long as she lived.

Cultural Elements of the Relationship Between the Individual and the Clinician

Because of the stigma associated with a mentally ill family member, Ms. B's husband initially attempted to treat her through consultation and medications provided by a colleague and social friend. She grew increasingly distrustful of her husband's motives and unconvinced about her actual need for treatment. She resisted treatment and saw it as a means for her husband to label her as crazy as a prelude to abandoning her. She was thus guarded about the intentions of the treating psychiatrist in this case, which created some difficulties initially in establishing and maintaining a working alliance.

Both the attending psychiatrist at the hospital and the treating psychiatrist during Ms. B's outpatient treatment were male, and both were interested and experienced in cultural psychiatry. A female nurse-clinician, who was about the patient's age, was her primary outpatient therapist for over 5 years. Neither the psychiatrist nor the nurse-clinician were of the same ethnic background as the patient and her husband, and these professionals were previously unknown to the B family. Care was taken by the psychiatrist and the nurse-clinician to avoid the perception of a collegial relationship with Dr. B throughout Ms. B's treatment. These elements proved helpful in establishing and maintaining a therapeutic alliance.

Overall Cultural Assessment for Diagnosis and Care

Faced with overwhelming stress in her family life and adaptation to living in the United States, Ms. B adopted a very traditional explanation of the misfortune that befell her and the children: that of malign magic induced by a jealous outsider. Her anger was thereby displaced from her husband to her sister-in-law, whom she accused first of overly influencing her husband and then of placing an evil spell that would bring misfortune and failure on them all. Such accusations further alienated her husband and ultimately led to her psychiatric admission. Her preoccupation with this explanation of her distress diminished over time, but it was never completely abandoned. However, another culturally accepted explanation took precedence; that of Fate or God's Will, which did not imply either shame or blame for Ms. B or her family. For psychotherapy to progress, it was necessary to take these heavily charged cultural factors into consideration. There was a complex interplay between the patient's intrapsychic vulnerabilities and the challenges of her environment that led to symptom formation, manifested in both personality features and severe existential concerns.

Clinical Course

Because of Ms. B's concerns about being mentally ill, her suspicions about her husband's motives, and her previous negative experiences with treatment and medication, treatment began with a discussion of her symptoms, her concerns, and the range of treatment options, in an attempt to ensure that she would experience the treatment as a collaborative process. The treating psychiatrist also agreed to use medications only as long as was necessary to bring her symptoms under control. Treatment with a combination of antipsychotic and antidepressant medication was recommended.[1] She refused the antidepressant (because of concerns about weight gain) and reluctantly agreed to take the antipsychotic medication. She was treated with perphenazine, 4 mg po in the morning and 8 mg po at bedtime, and benztropine, 2 mg po at bedtime. Restlessness, agitation, pressured speech, and paranoid ideations subsided in a short period of time, and medications were gradually reduced with no exacerbation of symptoms.

In individual psychotherapy Ms. B explored her feelings about her life experiences in Pakistan and over the past 20 years in the United States, her relationship with her husband, and her aspirations for herself

---

[1] The treatment took place before the newer generations of antipsychotic and antidepressant drugs came into use.

and her family. She was able to get in touch with her deep sense of lone-liness and isolation during the first few years in the United States, far from her family, friends, and Pakistani culture. As a newly married woman she had longed for the companionship that was absent because of her hus-band's busy surgical residency schedule. With the birth of her children she felt increasingly overburdened, isolated, and unsupported. She felt that her husband, who seemed to be adapting very well, opposed her as-pirations: to be more independent in the community, to continue her own education, and to take courses at a community college to improve her fluency in English and then perhaps do part-time work or volunteer community service. She was able to talk about her sense of inadequacy and her reluctance to assert herself, fearful of failure. She was also seen in daily group therapy sessions during her stay in the hospital and by weekly couple or family sessions. During family therapy sessions, the children were able to talk about their own aspirations for the future and their feelings about living in Pakistan as compared with the United States.

At the time of discharge Ms. B felt a greater sense of empowerment and hopefulness. There were no ideas of reference, and she did not want to hurt herself or family members. The strain in the relationship with her husband had subsided. She felt that treatment had been helpful and that her fears about being overmedicated had not materialized. She agreed to continue taking medications, which at time of discharge had been re-duced to perphenazine, 4 mg po at bedtime and benztropine, 1 mg po at bedtime. She remained somewhat depressed in mood, with low self-esteem, but she still refused antidepressant medication. She agreed, how-ever, to follow-up treatment with an experienced nurse-clinician, as well as continuing supervision of treatment by the attending psychiatrist.

For the next 5 years Ms. B continued in outpatient treatment, individ-ual psychotherapy, and couples' therapy. During the first year she was seen biweekly for 6 months, then every 3–4 weeks. In subsequent years the frequency of appointments varied with the circumstances and stress-ors in her life. Although her need for maintenance medication was clear, compliance remained a constant issue. When taking the medication, she was not preoccupied with being victimized by an evil spell perpetrated by her sister-in-law, and she complained much less about her husband's ignoring her opinions and feelings. Her mood was generally calmer, and she was less irritable and defensive. She was concerned, however, that her husband would disregard her issues and interpret any disagreement between them as the result of her not taking her medication or her need-ing a higher dose.

During the course of Ms. B's treatment the problems the children were experiencing became prominent. With individual psychotherapy the older daughter was able to remain in college and to complete her undergraduate degree without interruption. The younger daughter experienced similar self-doubts and adjustment problems when she started college 2 years later and, unlike the older sister, had to withdraw from college. She returned the following year and completed her undergraduate degree at a less prestigious college closer to home.

The family remained in crisis as problems emerged with the sons. The older son's behavior deteriorated during his high school years. He began to get into difficulties at school for being rowdy, cutting classes, and drinking. His grades declined sharply, and it was rumored that he was using drugs. Soon thereafter he started taking the car without permission, stealing money from home, and running up big expenses on his parents' credit cards. He was involved in several car accidents. He refused to comply with his parents' expectations and restrictions and became disrespectful and rebellious. He ignored and ridiculed their attempts to get him to stop his outrageous behavior. His previous enthusiasm for his father's life as a doctor rapidly declined. Although Dr. B initially made light of his son's problems, their seriousness became evident when his parents learned that he had lied about having taken his college entrance exams.

The problems with the younger son were even worse than with the older. After repeated incidents of disruptiveness and using alcohol and street drugs at school, he was expelled during his junior year. No other private school would accept him. He went to the local high school the following year, but his disruptive behavior continued. In the meantime, the older son was accepted at a local community college, but he failed again. At that point, he accepted the need for psychiatric help.

The problems in the marital relationship between Ms. B and her husband increased as the children's functioning deteriorated. Dr. B blamed the children's difficulties on Ms. B's unstable emotional condition. Ms. B's anger at her husband and the children grew intense. She felt helplessness and a sense of failure and despair. She needed to be seen more frequently in therapy to help her cope throughout the crises. In therapy she began to understand her loneliness and isolation in trying to live up to her husband's expectations (ever since they came to the United States), as well as how the expectations she and her husband had for their children were unrealistic. She realized that she and her husband could not impose their will on the children, that she was not responsible for their children's actions, and that the children had to learn from their own mistakes. She was then able to accept that she and her husband would have to cope with these family misfortunes as best they could, without mutual recriminations.

As Ms. B progressed in treatment, she became more self-confident and able to set boundaries, and she refused to accept full responsibility for everyone, their needs, and their behavior. When her mother-in-law had a stroke and her husband wanted to bring his mother to live with them, Ms. B refused to accept the arrangement. The expectation that she would nurse and look after her mother-in-law in their house, in addition to trying to cope with their two sons' rebellious behavior, was too much for her. Although Dr. B was angry and felt humiliated at being unable to fulfill his obligations to his sick and elderly mother, in the end he relented. That change in Dr. B led to a great decrease in the couple's mutual recriminations, and their coping abilities improved.

Ms. B continued to cope and to function without the need for rehospitalization during this 5-year period. Her treatment ended after the older daughter's marriage to a fellow student from an Arab country whom she had met during her senior year at college. The large wedding ceremony was a major event for the family and in the life of the whole Muslim community in the region.

Discussion

This case illustrates the complex interplay of biological and genetic vulnerability, personality structure, and the psychosocial factors related to familial strain and the effects of prolonged acculturative stress. Although disputed by the patient, there is evidence suggesting that Ms. B's mother was emotionally unstable and may have experienced one psychotic episode as an adult. The patient's life history was characterized by disruptions of security and affection that undermined the consolidation of her self-esteem and ego adaptive capacities. Her early years (0–9) were secure and stable, reinforcing a positive, confident sense of self and self-esteem. She described a nonstressful, financially and emotionally secure upbringing. The massive disruption and turmoil that attended the birth of India and Pakistan shattered this personal security. She was separated from her family during the civic turmoil in Pakistan and placed in a massive displacement camp for 6 months (9–10 years old) before being reunited with them. This left her with a vulnerability to loss, a fear of abandonment, and a sense of inadequacy. She thus always felt insecure, anxious, and vulnerable in her relationships.

The prominent defenses in her personality structure were splitting, displacement, and projection. Her parents, her sisters, and later her children were the idealized objects; her mother-in-law and sisters-in-law were the bad, demonized objects. Ms. B related to her husband as an ambivalently held object whom she experienced as supportive and affectionate, yet demeaning and tormenting. The idealization of objects (e.g., her parents, siblings, and husband) can be understood as a defense against rejection and abandonment. As a child separated from her family in war, she wished to blame her parents for her misfortune, but as a child she still needed to preserve an idealized image of them. Projection and displacement onto a readily available demonized enemy that could be blamed for the disasters and its associated emotional trauma also served to preserve the idealized image of her parents. These kinds of experiences in the early life of a child lay a psychological groundwork for subsequent splitting as a defense against loss and trauma as well as for a tendency toward idealization and devaluation.

Following the reunion with her family at age 10, the patient had a long period of restored security and accomplishment lasting through her teenage years and into early adulthood. During those years she completed high school and nursing training, was married, and set off for the United States with her husband for what she expected would be a 4- to 5-year stay before returning to the security of her family and homeland in Pakistan. Her old vulnerabilities resurfaced, however, as she gradually relinquished all the securities she had come to rely on and as she struggled to cope with demands of her husband's medical training in a strange and unfamiliar country and community, with little emotional support from him. She was flooded with sadness, loneliness, feelings of social isolation, and anger. The expression of her anger through accusations about her husband's behavior, which he strongly denied, led to increasing strain and emotional distance in the marital relationship, further undermining her sense of security and self-esteem.

The couple's marital relationship was further eroded by the patient's ongoing conflicts with her in-laws because of differing expectations and codes of behavior. She felt threatened by her husband's involvement with, and what she considered to be excessive obligation to, his family of origin and his disregard and neglect of her and the children. His ridicule, rejection, and humiliation of her further convinced her of his anticipated betrayal and ultimate abandonment. She attempted to contain her anxiety and intense anger through displacement: it was the sister-in-law who had put an evil spell on her that would bring misfortune to her, her children, and even her husband.

The patient's emotional turmoil and the strains in the marital relationship created tremendous difficulties and conflicts in the couple's ongoing attempts to adapt to the new culture while maintaining a sense of continuity with their culture of origin. This family—in turmoil and strained by the acculturative stress—was unable to provide an environment facilitating the acculturation and adaptation of their children. Thus the children became the bearers of the family's turmoil as they acted out and were unable to cope with normal developmental tasks in adolescence and early adulthood. This left the family in perpetual crisis until, with treatment, the patient was able to regain a sense of security and the couple was able to come together without mutual recriminations and with more realistic expectations of themselves, each other, and their children.

Asian Indians in the United States

Immigration of Indians and Pakistanis grew rapidly after passage of the Immigration and Naturalization Act of 1965. The 1990 United States census included more than 800,000 people of Asian Indian descent. Ten years later that number exceeded 2.2 million (U.S. Bureau of the Census 2000). Precise data are not available on the percentage distribution of Muslims among United States citizens of Indian or Pakistani heritage nor on the specific number of Pakistani Muslim immigrants in the United States (Almeida 1996; Williams 1991). It is clear, however, that Pakistani immigration has increased since the 1950s, particularly in the last decade, which saw an average rate of more than 10,000 new immigrants per year (Asian Migration News 2000). Among the distinguishing characteristics of these Asian Indian immigrants is that most of them are not refugees who have left their countries because of war or natural disaster. Large numbers have come to the United States in pursuit of advanced-level education and specialized training (Balagopal 1995; Leonhard-Spark et al. 1980). Another distinguishing feature of Asian Indians is their enormous diversity of racial groups, ethnicity, social class, religion, caste, and language, to the extent that overgeneralization is always a danger. However, it is helpful, in trying to understand the contextual cultural details of the B family case history, to describe some of the key features of Pakistani Muslim families who are immigrants to the United States.

Family structure is strongly patrilineal, patriarchal, and patrilocal. The patriarchal authority pattern includes respect for elders and loyalty to authority figures. The oldest male in the family retains decision-making authority for his children and grandchildren. In this type of patrilineal family structure, women have decidedly less status and authority than men, but there is still an age gradient for authority and respect, and the authority of mothers-in-law over their daughters-in-law and the grandchildren is legendary. The accomplishments—and failures—of all members of the family reflect on the reputation and status of the family. The actions of all family members can bring honor, as well as shame and dishonor, on the entire family (Ullrich 1997; Williams 1991).

Muslim religious observance requires individuals to adhere to strict codes of behavior involving dietary restrictions, avoidance of alcohol, prayers at prescribed times each day, and maintaining age- and sex-appropriate interactions with others. Men are constrained from interacting with women who are not relatives. Women's roles are expected to be confined largely to the home, and they are supposed to avoid interaction with men who are not from the immediate family. Premarital dating and sexual relationships are considered unacceptable. The developmental life stages of adolescence and early adulthood did not exist until recently and have been a source of great turmoil for parents and children, since there has been no tradition of youth experimenting with dating relationships, making career choices, or selecting marriage partners. Marriages were approved and arranged by parents for the benefit of the entire family (Almeida 1996; Ullrich 1997).

The potential for intrafamilial conflict among Pakistani Muslim immigrants to the United States is great, given the existing sharp differences in expectations of appropriate social behavior. Maintaining close contact with "home" in Pakistan through telecommunication links and regular visits can itself intensify intrafamilial conflict, even as it helps the family members reinforce cultural identity and maintain emotional connections with family and friends. It is quite possible that maintaining close contact of this kind engenders ambivalence toward both cultures. That is, the immigrants' life in the United States is usually a source of status and prestige to the family when they visit Pakistan but also engenders envy and resentment at the erosion of the accustomed deference to authority and traditional ways of doing things. On the other hand, when the immigrants are living in the United States, they tend to idealize their preimmigration life in Pakistan and expect it to be unchanged, familiar, and accepting of them as unchanged too when they return to visit. In this way, frustration and dissatisfaction with their life in one country enhances their idealization of and denial of problems in living in the other country (Ullrich 1997).

In the process of adapting to life in the United States, the children of immigrants grow up with a much greater exposure to American norms of social interaction and inevitably are strongly influenced by youth culture as encountered in school. For children born in the United States, the potential for intergenerational conflict about values and social behavior is particularly high. It has led to the popularized term of "ABCDs" to describe this group: American Born Confused Deshis (nationals) (Ullrich 1997; Williams 1991).

The case of the B family eloquently illustrates acculturation as a journey of discovery that can—and often does—engender a great deal of stress. Separation from the larger community was the predominant but not the only direction of adaptation to acculturative stress for both Ms. B and her husband. As with so many people faced with complex adaptations, outcomes were influenced not only by their own wishes but by those of their family members and by the impinging pressures of the outside world. Dr. and Ms. B's wishes for separation were in conflict with their own and their children's aspirations for closer interaction with the larger community. Nevertheless, the older generation's predominant orientation was toward psychological separation and remained so, despite the intrapsychic and intrafamilial conflicts it generated. In turn, marginalization was the direction of acculturative stress most descriptive of the chaotic stage of both sons' adolescent and early adult years. The two daughters had shown some evidence of going in the same direction, but they managed to regain some psychological balance and perspective through a period of psychosocial moratorium and, in the case of the older daughter, through the assistance of psychotherapy.

The literature on acculturation emphasizes the need for long-term study of the process. The outcome of acculturative stress, as demonstrated by the case of Ms. B's family, cannot be understood by cross-sectional, short-term analysis. The process is continuous throughout the life cycle and is strongly influenced by events over which individuals, families, and communities have little control. At the same time, understanding the theoretical underpinnings of acculturative stress and its psychological outcome can enable clinicians to take account of its complex influence on the clinical presentation of the large number of people affected by it. Clinicians can thereby improve the quality of their treatment.

■ References

Almeida R: Hindu, Christian and Muslim families, in Ethnicity and Family Therapy. Edited by McGoldrick M, Giordano ZJ, Pearce JK. New York, Guilford Press, 1996, pp 121–133

Asian Migration News: http://www.scalabrini.org/~smc/amnews/amnews1.htm. Retrieved from the World Wide Web 5/3/2000

Balagopal PR: Asian Indians, in Encyclopedia of Social Work. Washington, DC, NASW Press, 1995, pp 615–616

Leonhard-Spark PJ, Saran P, Ginsberg K: The Indian immigrant in America: a demographic profile, in The New Ethnics: The Case of South Asian Indians Edited by Saram P, Eames E. New York, Praeger, 1980, pp 136–149

Ullrich HE: Breaking the cultural barrier: issues for psychotherapy among Indian immigrants. Paper presented at the Second National Asian-Indian American Conference: Exploration and Identity, Rutgers University, New Brunswick, NJ, 1997

U.S. Bureau of the Census: Economics and Statistics Administration. Washington, DC, U.S. Department of Commerce, 1993

Williams R: Asian-Indian Muslims in the United States, in Indian Muslims in North America. Edited by Khalidi O. Watertown, MA, South Asia Press, 1991

■ An Asian American Student's Reticence

A Filipino American medical student cannot speak in class for fear that she will be criticized and humiliated. She postpones dealing with this and other personal issues during college in order to focus on her goal of being admitted to medical school. Once she begins medical school, she realizes that it is time to address her speaking anxiety, since she will soon be required to give regular presentations on hospital rounds. She goes to a student counseling office and asks to be seen by a female Asian American clinician.

This case demonstrates the usefulness of the DSM-IV-TR Outline for Cultural Formulation (American Psychiatric Association 2000, Appendix I), which led to a more thorough understanding of the various factors contributing to the patient's anxiety. The cultural formulation also provides a springboard for a richer understanding of the patient's inner dynamics, presenting fields of exploration that would have been unseen if culture were not considered.

Special considerations in the diagnosis and treatment of social phobia in Asian Americans are addressed. This is an especially pertinent topic, given the overlap between symptoms of this disorder and normal culturally appropriate behavior in many Asian cultures. Finally, the case raises questions about the larger sociocultural implications of diagnosing and treating social phobia in Asian Americans.

Identifying Data

Ms. C was a 24-year-old single Asian American female medical student who was born in the Philippines and who immigrated with her family to the United States when she was 6 years old.

Reason for Evaluation

Throughout high school and college, Ms. C had coped with her public speaking anxiety by avoiding it. Knowing that avoidance would no longer be possible when she would be required to give presentations on hospital rounds, she knew that it was time to seek help.

History of Present Illness

Ms. C stated that her anxiety about speaking in class was so severe that, to the best of her recollection, she had never done it. She feared that professors and peers would call her stupid and that they would humiliate her, make her an outcast, and eventually ostracize her from school. Sometimes she would become so anxious she would feel dizzy.

She had known since her early college years that she had a problem. However, she postponed seeking help in order to focus on getting good grades so that she could be admitted to medical school. She reached her objective, but during her first semester there she became so disturbed about her public-speaking anxiety that she stopped attending classes. She felt extremely depressed and hated herself. She felt lethargic, slept too much, and had frequent crying spells. At one point she did not leave her home for 2 weeks. There were no thoughts of suicide, but this was the first time Ms. C had been so depressed that it interfered in a significant manner with her functioning. These symptoms resolved spontaneously within 8 weeks while Ms. C was on a Christmas vacation.

During the second semester Ms. C decided to seek help, realizing that in order to complete medical school she would need to speak in front of others. She was especially concerned that during her third year she would need to make presentations regularly in different settings and practically all the time. She went to the Student Counseling Center and requested help, stating that she preferred to be seen by a female Asian American clinician. She felt that an Asian American might have an understanding of the aspects of her personality and values that she attributed to her Asian cultural upbringing. She also felt that an Asian American therapist would be less likely to see her problems as weird.

At the time of the evaluation, her depressive symptoms and crying spells had resolved and her energy and sleep patterns had returned to normal. However, her anxiety about speaking in class and her low self-esteem related to this matter remained unchanged. In addition, Ms. C complained of other related problems, such as difficulty in asserting herself in laboratory groups, especially when it would involve contradicting classmates. For example, during one laboratory assignment, Ms. C's group had decided to proceed in a manner that she knew would fail. However, she could not bring herself to tell them. After her group had gone through multiple failures, Ms. C finally expressed her ideas on how to handle the project. They followed her suggestions, and their next attempt was successful. According to Ms. C, she would never want to assume a leadership position from the start. However, if for some reason it was necessary for her to do so, then she would do it for the good of the group.

Ms. C also experienced anxiety in a variety of other social situations.

She envied the way some of her classmates would have casual conversations with her professors. Whenever she would see a professor by chance at school, she would either go to great lengths to avoid him or her, or she would make a quick greeting and then scurry away. Ms. C realized that she felt especially uncomfortable in small groups led by a male professor, and she wished she could "chum" with her professors the way her classmates did. At lunchtime, she usually ate with one of her classmates, another Asian American woman. When this classmate was unavailable, she ate alone, all the while feeling anxious about others observing her doing so. Ms. C would join others only if asked, since she would not want to intrude upon them otherwise. A similar anxiety would occur at parties, when she would be very anxious about socializing. She would sit with her boyfriend and join others only when asked. Often she would go home wondering why she bothered to go to parties.

Past Psychiatric History

This was Ms. C's first contact with a mental health care professional. Actually, it can be said that her past psychiatric history weaves into the history of her present illness.

General Medical History

Ms. C had no significant medical history, was taking no medications, and had no known drug allergies.

Ms. C used alcohol rarely, and she had never tried any illegal substances.

Developmental History

Ms. C was born in the Philippines and moved with her family to the United States when she was 6 years old. She was the youngest of four children. Her father, a man in his late fifties, worked as a supervisor in a local government agency. Her mother, a woman in her early fifties, worked in a factory. Ms. C had three older siblings: two sisters and a brother. All were within 6 years of her age, were college graduates with some graduate education, and had successful professional careers. Their father had decided that the family should emigrate to the United States, as he thought opportunities for his children would be greater. The family had moved to a suburban community in California and had lived there ever since.

Adjusting to life in the United States was difficult for Ms. C's father, who started drinking heavily and became irritable at home. Ms. C recalls once asking at the dinner table how to say a certain word in Tagalog. Her father became angry that his children had forgotten how to speak Tagalog and raged that from then on, only Tagalog could be spoken in the house. After he left the dinner table, her siblings criticized her for having asked this question. At another time she asked her father to help with her homework. He became angry and called her stupid. She never asked him for help again. In retrospect, she realized that he had probably felt inadequate to help her and that he was being defensive. She suspected that her relationship with her father might be related to her anxiety about speaking in class.

Her mother was a nurturing and consistent figure in the family's life. She would often dissipate her husband's anger and smooth over potential or actual conflicts. Her devotion to her family was illustrated in one of Ms. C's recurring dreams. In this dream, Ms. C and her mother would hide behind the living room sofa, dodging enemy gunfire. Sometimes her mother would leave their sofa foxhole to walk toward the kitchen. She would get shot, and Ms. C would run out and hold her bleeding mother in her arms. Then her mother would get up and continue toward the kitchen to prepare dinner for her family. This scenario would repeat itself continuously.

Ms. C states that her parents put pressure on her oldest sister to go to medical school and become a doctor. However, she did not excel enough academically and became a pharmacist instead. Ms. C stated that she did not believe the other children underwent the same parental pressures as her oldest sister did. All, however, were far better educated than their parents.

Ms. C lived at home during her first 2 years of college, then transferred to a more prestigious university away from home for the remainder of her studies. As another sister lived near the university, Ms. C moved in with her. They shared cooking and cleaning chores. At the time of presentation, Ms. C had never lived independently.

Ms. C had met her boyfriend when they were both age 16. He was Caucasian American, and they attended the same high school. Following high school, he worked in the computer field; he had never attended college. According to Ms. C, this discrepancy in their educational levels was disturbing to him but not to her. They had a supportive relationship, and Ms. C found him comforting when she felt distressed about her difficulties at school.

Social History

Ms. C felt guilty about having moved away from home even though she recognized the necessity for it. She worried that her parents were lonely and sad without their children at home, particularly as she was the last child to leave. She and her sister had frequent contact with their parents by phone and visited them almost every weekend. Often these visits would occur when their mother asked them to come home and do domestic chores. Ms. C believed her mother used the chores as a way of asking her children to visit and that the chores themselves were not important. This was a source of conflicting feelings for Ms. C: as she became busier with medical school, she felt increasingly burdened by visiting her parents so regularly. When she began her clinical rotations, she would have few free weekends, and she did not want to spend them working at her parents' home.

Occupational History

During the first summer of medical school, Ms. C did research as part of a fellowship she had earned. Other than this, she had never been employed and was financially supported by her parents.

Family History

Ms. C's parents had met and married in the Philippines, where her father belonged to a large family working mostly in manual and field labor. His family considered him unusual because he felt education was important, and when he earned his bachelor's degree, his family failed to attend his graduation. According to Ms. C, the desire for his children to be educated was a main factor in her father's decision to emigrate.

When Ms. C's family came to the United States, her father became separated from relatives and lifelong friends. According to Ms. C, her father was popular and well connected in the Philippines. Whenever he returned to visit, there would be many parties welcoming him. Through his government connections he was able to help relatives get jobs in the Philippines, even though he lived in the United States. In the Philippines, her father often drank socially with groups of male friends, but in the United States he no longer had this group of friends, so he drank alone. Ms. C recalls him drinking shots of hard liquor in the morning, before afternoon naps, and after dinner. She believed that all the men she knew in the Philippines drank but that the stresses of dislocation probably caused her father to drink more heavily and even excessively. He had no history of treatment for this drinking problem.

While her family lived in the Philippines, her older brother was treated by a "witch doctor." He was about 10 years old, and it was believed that he was possessed. Ms. C remembered her mother burying items beneath a mango tree as part of his treatment. In adulthood, her brother underwent psychotherapy in the United States. However, Ms. C did not believe that he was treated with medication. She did not know the nature of the symptoms for which he sought treatment.

Review of Systems

A review of systems revealed only the dizziness that often accompanied her anxiety episodes.

Physical Examination

The physical examination was deferred, because Ms. C was seen as an outpatient and because she had no significant medical history or physical complaints.

Mental Status Examination

Ms. C was a petite woman who looked younger than her age. She was always neatly groomed and wore casual, inconspicuous clothing, such as jeans and shirts in shades of brown and tan. She wore glasses with large plastic frames that hid her face. She wore no makeup. She appeared anxious in the first interview, but in subsequent sessions she showed a more relaxed demeanor. Her speech was of normal rhythm, rate, and volume. She was articulate and quite verbally expressive.

Ms. C described herself as usually being a happy-go-lucky person and denied any chronic mood symptoms. Indeed, she was usually bright, cheerful, and congenial, but she expressed self-deprecating feelings in regard to her inability to speak in class. Her thoughts were coherent and of normal form and content. There was no history of psychotic symptoms and no history of suicidal ideation. She was alert, with a clear sensorium, and seemed to function at a high intellectual level with good cognitive abilities. Memory and ability to abstract were excellent. She had a good fund of knowledge and appeared to have excellent judgment. She also appeared to have a good amount of psychological insight.

At the time of evaluation, there were no vegetative symptoms of depression such as sleep or appetite disturbance, nor were there symptoms consistent with a history of mania, such as periods of increased energy or decreased need for sleep.

Functional Assessment

Ms. C functioned at a high level and had earned good grades and a fellowship in medical school. Socially, she also functioned well, having supportive relationships with her family and her long-term boyfriend. Her social anxiety, however, interfered with her performance at school as well as with relationships with peers. In the context of medical school, there was a significant impairment whenever she was required to speak in front of others.

Diagnostic Tests

Routine laboratory values were within normal limits. They included thyroid function tests, complete blood count, electrolytes, liver function tests, and urinalysis.

DSM-IV-TR Diagnosis

Axis I
Social phobia
Academic problem
Major depression, single episode, moderate, in full remission
Rule out acculturation problem

Axis II
None

Axis III
None

Axis IV
Acute stressor: requirements to speak in medical school
Chronic stressor: negotiating between the Asian culture of her home environment and the American culture of school and society at large

Axis V
   GAF pretreatment=65
   GAF posttreatment=85

Differential Diagnosis

Under the conventional DSM-IV-TR diagnostic system, Ms. C met full criteria for the diagnosis of social phobia: her anxiety about speaking in front of others, her fear of negative evaluation, her own recognition that her fear was excessive, the anxiety interfering with her performance in medical school, the persistence of this anxiety for all of her years of schooling, and her avoidance of anxiety-provoking social situations such as speaking in class.

Other anxiety disorders were considered and excluded, as her anxiety was limited to social performance situations. She experienced dizziness but no other physical symptoms of anxiety. Therefore, she did not meet criteria for panic attacks or panic disorder. There was no clear history of trauma, which would be essential for the diagnosis of posttraumatic stress disorder. In fact, she seemed to have managed appropriately her father's unpredictable behavior, even though she attributed at least part of her anxiety symptoms to such factor.

The diagnosis of adjustment disorder with anxious and depressed mood was excluded because of the long-standing nature of Ms. C's problem. Before the evaluation, Ms. C had undergone an episode of depression, which lasted less than 8 weeks and which prevented her from attending class or even leaving her home for 2 weeks. This episode had apparently resolved spontaneously.

Other mood disorders were considered. Ms. C had never experienced symptoms consistent with mania. The possibility of chronic dysthymia was also dismissed, since her discontent was limited to school-related performance situations. On weekends, she enjoyed herself with her boyfriend, friends, and siblings.

There was no evidence of a personality disorder. Her avoidance was limited to social performance situations, and she never avoided school or family responsibilities. She had a stable relationship with her boyfriend of 8 years.

Cultural Formulation

Cultural Identity of the Individual

Ms. C was born in the Philippines and considered herself an American. She has a Spanish first name and surname and chooses friends who are Asian American, not necessarily of Filipino heritage. None of this should be considered unusual. Historical and cultural factors contributing to the complexity of her Filipino American identity will be addressed in the Discussion section.

Cultural Explanations of the Individual's Symptoms

Within the context of many Asian cultures, Ms. C's anxieties and behaviors would not be considered outside the range of normal. Three concepts central to many Asian and Asian American cultures should be taken into account whenever considering the diagnosis of social phobia in an Asian American: 1) The concept of "face" and the importance of not losing it; 2) respect for elders, a deeply rooted value in Asian cultures; and 3) group-oriented thinking, which is a norm in Asian and Asian American cultures rather than the rugged individualism that is so stressed in mainstream American culture. In the Philippines, two terms reflecting this belief are *pakakisama* (the value of conceding to the wishes of the group) and *kapwa* (the concept of shared identity).

Cultural Factors Related to Psychosocial Environment and Levels of Functioning

Many of Ms. C's anxieties reflected culturally appropriate values in Filipino, Chinese, and other Asian cultures. For example, her anxiety about being humiliated in class was consistent with the preoccupation with "saving face." Her reticence about having casual conversations with professors reflected the value of respect for elders. Her reserve about assuming leadership reflected her valuing *pakakisama*. With her laboratory group, Ms. C deferred to the wishes of the group, whereas other group members were more aggressive and assertive, as might be expected in the culture of an American medical school. Much of Ms. C's discomfort in group situations also reflected her cultural dislocation, since group etiquette in Asian and American cultures differs. For example, during the times she ate lunch alone, if she had been in an Asian cultural setting, someone eating with a group might ask Ms. C to join them, as part *of kapwa*. Overall, Ms. C was behaving in ways appropriate to Asian culture.

However, she was trying to function in the aggressive psychosocial environment of an American medical school.

Cultural Elements of the Relationship Between the
Individual and the Clinician

On a very basic level, Ms. C and the therapist shared many cultural commonalities, because both were Asian American, sharing the experience of being Asian, and therefore different, in America. This was true even though Ms. C's ancestry, from the tropical islands of the Philippines, differed in many respects, from the therapist's ancestry in the mountains of snowy northern China. Although distinct and heterogeneous, Chinese, Filipino, and other Asian cultures often have such commonalities. Ms. C and the therapist also shared the common experiences of immigrating to the United States at a young age in the post-1965 Asian immigration wave, following the lifting of anti-Asian immigration quotas.

Ms. C requested an Asian American therapist out of the fear that someone who was not Asian American might think her "weird." The therapist found Ms. C's anxieties quite understandable, having had many Asian American patients, friends, and relatives with similar perspectives and similar problems.

Of interest also is that both the patient and the therapist had Latin roots within their cultural backgrounds: Spain has had centuries of influence upon Filipino culture, and the therapist's family was Chinese-Brazilian—her mother was mostly raised in Brazil, where her family had settled after the civil war in China. The therapist was born in Brazil, and during most of her childhood in the United States, her family thought of Brazil as home. The convergence of backgrounds is an example of the fluid nature of culture and the increasingly blurred boundaries between cultural identities today.

Overall Cultural Assessment for Diagnosis and Care

Although Ms. C exhibited many symptoms which met criteria for social phobia, it was also apparent that she was constantly negotiating between the Asian cultural values of her home and family and the more American values of her school environment. This was made evident throughout the cultural assessment.

Not only were Ms. C and her family separated from relatives and friends in the Philippines, they were also enduring the stress of constantly negotiating between cultures. She not only had to cope with her own losses but also absorbed the unhappiness of her parents. For example, her father had endured the loss of family, close friends, a familiar way of life, and an influential social status. The losses and trauma of the parent generation can be transmitted to children, who must compensate for the anxieties of their parents. Often these children incur double losses, as they not only lose the nurturing of their parents but also must give comfort to soothe their parents' anxieties.

Clinical Course

Treatment consisted of weekly psychotherapy, which addressed issues of adjustment and focused most prominently on Ms. C's social phobia symptoms as the most pressing issue. Cognitive-behavioral techniques targeting social phobia symptoms as well as psychodynamic approaches to exploring adjustment issues were employed. Through the course of cognitive-behavioral therapy, Ms. C realized that her automatic thoughts consisted of cognitive distortions, such as jumping to conclusions that she would be criticized, seeing things through a mental filter portraying everything in a negative light, and catastrophizing: thinking that small errors would result in far-reaching consequences, such as failing school and being ostracized by her peers. Ms. C began to recognize her cognitive distortions; she began to make brief comments in class and to be able to participate in small-group discussions. However, she still had significant anxiety about speaking up in front of larger groups.

Ms. C's treatment became urgent when she was asked to present her summer research project at a national conference. She realized that this was an honor, since most presenters would be faculty, and few students were invited. However, the prospect of standing next to her poster and answering questions for several hours seemed insurmountable. In addition, she was anxious about traveling alone to an unfamiliar city. In the past when had she traveled alone, she had avoided contact with people and isolated herself in her hotel room. She strongly considered refusing the invitation.

At this point, antianxiety medications were discussed. Ms. C agreed to a trial of propranolol, 10 mg po before social performance situations. Her first use was during a lecture in a large classroom. To her surprise, when she thought of a question, she quickly raised her hand and asked it. Her question was well received, and classmates complimented her afterward.

She attended the conference. With the use of propranolol, she presented her poster without difficulty. She also enjoyed a party without her usual anxiety and reticence. She went to a restaurant and enjoyed eating lunch alone. At another point, she telephoned student presenters from other medical schools and organized an outing. Toward the end of the conference, she volunteered to participate in a panel discussion and did so without the use of propranolol. Ms. C returned home satisfied that not only had she successfully presented her research, but that she had made new friends.

When she returned to school, she continued to participate regularly in classes without the use of the medication. When clinical rotations began, Ms. C started with 8 weeks of surgery. She completed the clerkship, regularly made presentations, and tolerated critical remarks from surgery attendings and house staff.

From the cultural perspective, Ms. C also resolved many issues with her family during the course of treatment. She realized that her inner turmoil about how much time she should spend with her family constituted retaining Filipino cultural ideals, but living in the reality of American culture. She realized that in the Philippines village where her family had lived, children would usually grow up and build homes in the same neighborhood as their parents. This would result in large extended family networks that had frequent contact. She realized that in the United States, most families lived differently, and children usually moved away from their parents. Moreover, given her situation, it would not have been possible for her to meet the same family expectations as she would if her family still lived in the village. She informed her mother of this insight and her mother received it well, pleased that Ms. C had been so concerned for the happiness of her parents.

At times the therapist tried to bring up other issues of culture with Ms. C. However, she usually seemed reluctant to discuss them. This was interpreted not as denial or avoidance but as her reticence about engaging in a discussion that seemed artificial. Just as a therapeutic dyad of Caucasian American therapist and patient would not need to dwell on issues of American culture, this therapeutic dyad did not need to overemphasize culture: cultural understanding was implicit during the sessions. However, the therapeutic relationship benefited from common understandings. For example, as an Asian American, the therapist was able to empathize with Ms. C's predicament about her loyalty to her parents, as well as her ambivalence in social situations.

When the decision to terminate therapy was made because Ms. C was beginning her busy clerkship year and because the therapist was planning on relocating to another state, the therapist asked Ms. C if she would like the therapist's new phone number should Ms. C need help. She declined. Instead, she requested a prescription for a small quantity of propranolol, which she had not used in approximately a year. Asking for the medicine was symbolic of Ms. C's desire to seek support only if she needed it. The therapist gave her the prescription and also the new phone number, understanding that Ms. C had originally refused it out of *pakakisama,* and perhaps even out of respect for the therapist as an elder, as well as her desire to not impose herself. Perhaps Ms. C thought that the therapist had originally offered the phone number also out of *pakakisama* and politeness. Later, however, she understood that the therapist's offer was heartfelt, and she took the phone number eagerly and appeared relieved. This type of exchange is typical among Asians and Asian Americans: one person may make an offer; the other refuses out of politeness. A round (or often several rounds) of offers and polite refusals will ensue as the two parties feel each other out. Each round allows the parties involved to discover empathetically what would be in the best interest of both involved. Each offer and refusal is highly symbolic, and more is at stake than simply goods or services. Each offer and refusal is an expression of one's desire to think of the other's welfare and to anticipate the other's needs. The good of the group is valued over an individual's wants. The wants of one person are not separable from the wants of others. A quite typical Asian and Asian American view is that what is best for the group is ultimately what is best for the individual as well.

Discussion

The following is a discussion of three values (face, respect for elders, and group-oriented thinking) common to many Asian and Asian American cultures. These values should be taken into account whenever the diagnosis of social phobia is considered in an Asian American patient. An assessment of other clinical and cultural issues of the case will follow.

Face

In Filipino culture this concept is called *hiya;* in Chinese culture it is called *lian*. It is often translated into English as *face,* although there is no real English equivalent. If one does something to shame oneself, it is said that one has "lost face." Great extremes will be endured in order to save face, as the loss of face may imply dire consequences.

Because of the strong cohesion of families, one person's shameful act may reflect on the entire family. Honor is important, and if an individual is shamed, then "both the individual and the family are placed in a position of *hiya* or loss of face" (Pido 1986, p. 45). An extreme example of the consequence of losing face would be to remove the shame from the family by removing oneself through the act of suicide. Whereas in Western cultures, suicide is considered a sin or a crime against society, it has a different connotation in Asian cultures: suicide may be viewed as an honorable way to save face and to save one's family from shame. In the United States, stories of Asian American students committing suicide over a bad grade are unfortunately not uncommon.

Although suicide is an extreme example of the lengths to which Asians will go to save face, it nevertheless emphasizes the gravity and importance of face in Asian cultures. For Asian American students, making an embarrassing comment in class or being criticized in class carries the additional monumental weight of possibly losing face. When considering the diagnosis of social phobia in an Asian American such as Ms. C, the importance of face must be taken into account.

Respect for Elders

This value is deeply ingrained in most Asian cultures, and it stands in stark contrast to the youth-oriented culture of the United States:

> Respect for the elder is one Filipino value that has remained in the book of unwritten laws. The Filipino parents exercise almost absolute powers over the children. It is unthinkable for a Filipino to do an important thing without consulting his parents. The language of the Filipino denotes deep-seated respect for elders especially in the use of the particle po [a term of respect used when addressing an elder]. (Andres 1981, p. 52)

Filial piety, an English phrase that can serve as an extraordinarily awkward translation of an Asian concept with no real Western equivalent today, governs parent-child relationships. Good sons and daughters are expected to be all-sacrificing toward their parents and to put the good of their parents above all, including career, spouse, and their own children. They should never argue with their parents or display rebelliousness. They should obey unquestioningly.

In the classroom, this concept of respect for elders applies to the teacher-student relationship. In Filipino culture, one uses the term of respect *po* when addressing an elder. One would never address a professor by a first name, as is common in the United States, and one would not behave in a familiar fashion with professors. In a traditional Chinese classroom, for example, students may often avoid eye contact with teachers as a sign of respect. Casual conversations do not occur. This traditional value of respecting elders explains much of Ms. C's socially reticent behavior toward her professors.

Group-Oriented Thinking

As noted previously, Filipinos value the concept of *pakakisama,* or conceding to the wishes of the group (Araneta 1993; Pido 1986). This complements the previously mentioned core Filipino value of *kapwa* (shared identity), which is considered at the foundation of human values, and without which one ceases to be Filipino and human (Strobel 1994). Chinese children are brought up with the concept of *hu xiang bang zu,* or group thinking and helpfulness. According to philosopher Tu Wei Min, in classical Confucian thought, the self is considered the sum of one's relationships, and one develops the self through interactions with others (Tu 1984).

Asians tend to function more as members of a group than as individuals separate from a group. The assertive individualism that is so valued in the United States has no place in many Asian cultures. Whereas Americans can view aggressiveness as a positive trait, Asians value humility and smooth interpersonal relationships with members of the group. In fact, if one acts overly confident and is later humiliated by failure, it would be a cause for loss of face for the individual and his or her family. A Filipino who is viewed as acting mostly in his or her own interest would be viewed with distrust and suspicion (Pido 1986). Ms. C deferred to others in her opinions when someone else assumed leadership, yet she was willing to assume leadership when no one else would. This reflects her priority to act in the best interest of the group and to preserve smooth interpersonal relationships. She was demonstrating the value of *pakakisama.*

Clinical Issues

Many scholars, including psychologists and literary writers, have explored a perceived social reserve among Asian Americans. A survey of Asian American college students found that more than 90% felt that members of their minority group should be more assertive. Moreover, they personally expressed interest in assertiveness training programs (Sue 1977). A study of social anxiety comparing Chinese American and Caucasian American women indicated that Chinese American women had a significantly higher fear of negative evaluation (Sue et al. 1989). Going from the sciences to literature, in her autobiographical novel *The Woman Warrior,* Maxine Hong Kingston writes: "When I went to kindergarten and had to speak English for the first time, I became silent. A dumbness—a shame—still cracks my voice in two....The other Chinese girls did not talk either, so I knew that the silence had to do with being a Chinese girl" (Kingston 1977, p. 62). In Ms. C's case, her family's migration story adds to the experience that Grinberg and Grinberg (1989) call "cumulative trauma," emphasizing that migration precipitates a series of ongoing and enduring stressors. As noted before, the concept of double losses also applies here as a pathogenic and pathoplastic element. Although it originated from studies of children of Holocaust survivors, double loss is a valuable theory with potentially widespread applications. It can be applied to children of parents who have endured significantly difficult circumstances such as the experience of migration (Brown and Shanahan 1995).

Is the incidence of social phobia higher in Asian Americans than in the general United States population? Studies of this topic have yet to be carried out. However, before exploring this question, it would be worthwhile to examine Asian American cultural values and judgments—that is, the elements of countertransference. As mental health care practitioners who apply the principles of psychiatry, psychology, and social sciences—with predominantly Western civilization roots—it is important to examine countertransference and cultural biases when passing judgment on other cultures. Does the whole concept of social phobia reflect Western ideals and Western concepts of mental health? In Asian cultures, where social interactions occur in a more structured fashion and where the fear of negative evaluation (or fear of losing face) may be an ingrained cultural value, is the concept of social phobia relevant?

Another important question concerns the implications of the changes Ms. C underwent in the course of her treatment for symptoms of social phobia. She became less fearful of being shamed in class, more willing to contradict teachers, and more independent and detached from her family. It can be argued that treatment enabled her to become less Asian and more American.

That psychiatry's role is to decrease discomfort caused by emotional conflicts is well accepted. However, the ethical implications of altering a patient's cultural values has yet to be extensively explored in the field of mental health.

In any case, Ms. C. benefited from the treatment of symptoms of social phobia, because the change resulting from her treatment enabled her to function more comfortably in American culture and because it allowed her to continue striving toward her goal of becoming a physician.

■ References

American Psychiatric Association: Diagnostic and Statistical Manual of Mental Disorders, 4th Edition, Text Revision. Washington, DC, American Psychiatric Association, 2000

Andres T: Understanding Filipino Values: A Management Approach. Quezon City, Philippines, New Day Publishers, 1981

Araneta E: Psychiatric Care of Pilipino Americans, in Culture, Ethnicity and Mental Illness. Edited by Gaw A. Washington, DC, American Psychiatric Press, 1993, pp 377–411

Brown EM, Shanahan K: A New Story of Healing: Breaking Through Silences of the "Double Losses" for the Second and Third Generations of Holocaust Families. Paper presented at the annual meeting of the American Society of Orthopsychiatry, April 1995

Grinberg L, Grinberg R: Psychoanalytic Perspectives on Migration and Exile. New Haven, CT, Yale University Press, 1989

Kingston MH: The Woman Warrior: Memoirs of a Girlhood Among Ghosts. New York, Vintage Books, 1977

Machida M: Addressing East/West Interaction, in Asia/America: Identities in Contemporary Asian American Art. The Asia Society Galleries, New York, New Press, 1994, pp 35–39

Pido AJA: The Pilipinos in America: Macro/Micro Dimensions of Immigration and Integration. New York, Center for Migration Studies, 1986

Strobel LM: Cultural identity of third-wave Filipino Americans. Journal of the American Association for Philippine Psychology 1:37–54, 1994

Sue D, Sue DM, Ino S: Assertiveness and Social Anxiety in Chinese-American Women. Psychology 124:155–163, 1989

Sue S: Psychological theory and implications for Asian Americans. Personnel and Guidance Journal 55:381–389, 1977

Takaki R: Strangers from a Different Shore: A History of Asian Americans. Boston, MA, Little, Brown, 1989

Tu WM: Confucian Ethics Today. Singapore City, Singapore Federal Publications, 1984

■ African Tribal Roots

This case offers examples of multiple losses, including loss of country of origin and family ties, as stressors leading to depressive symptoms. The case also deals with issues of immigration and acculturation, including the part played by religious or spiritual problems in the origin of psychopathology and the use of religious ritual as a means of reparation. Diagnostically, this case illustrates the application of the DSM-IV-TR Outline for Cultural Formulation to an inpatient treatment, using an understanding of the role of culture in obtaining compliance and in the development of rapport between the patient and the treatment team. The case also explores

- The cultural conflicts of interracial marriage
- The role played by family/community networks
- Gender roles as manifestations of cultural norms
- Issues of drug abuse and self-medication
- The importance of religious rituals in healing and reestablishing broken relationships
- The relevance of a client-directed model, as demonstrated by the patient actively participating in his own treatment planning

The case also highlights the cultural competence required of the multidisciplinary treatment team in order to 1) apply culturally syntonic interventions and 2) identify culturally relevant outpatient programs and community networks to enhance the quality of follow-up care.

Identifying Data

Mr. D was a 30-year-old heterosexual African Kikuyu tribesman from Kenya, born and raised as a Catholic, with some college background and English as a second language. He had married, 11 years before coming to treatment, a white American woman working in Africa as a Catholic missionary. He immigrated to the United States with his wife and three children (ages 10, 8, and 6) 9 years before coming to treatment and had been working cleaning furniture until shortly before beginning treatment. Five days prior to admission, he left his job and house and began living in his pickup truck. This was his first psychiatric experience.

Reason for Evaluation

Mr. D was brought in to a hospital emergency room by the state Highway Patrol after he left a bridge, where he had contemplated killing himself. He reported that while on the bridge he decided to call the suicide hotline and subsequently was on 72-hour involuntary commitment for evaluation.

History of Present Illness

The patient stated that he had been using crack cocaine for the past 3 years and had used crystal methamphetamine for several years before that. He had kept his drug use secret from his wife, knowing that she would object. Recently, his wife had become suspicious when she discovered that he was spending $200 a day. In the course of time he felt the need to confide in her but feared confrontation and marital disharmony. During Catholic confession, he was instructed to "tell everything." His wife became angry and questioned his faithfulness. She decided to leave home, taking the three children with her. Nevertheless, he continued to use crack cocaine. His business finally collapsed as well. He felt depressed during the day, then he would smoke cocaine and feel better only to become depressed again—"a roller coaster ride." He would also occasionally smoke marijuana to "calm down." Recently, he had started contemplating killing himself. He had squandered $12,000 of family savings within a period of 7 weeks. In the 2 weeks prior to this hospitalization, Mr. D had made serious suicidal plans: "I doused the garage with gasoline but didn't light it. I had an office in the garage where I would smoke crack….I wanted to burn the cave [as he called his office]. I left and never returned to the house afterward." He had also attempted to hang himself with a rope in the cellar; this attempt was unsuccessful, as the wooden beam broke.

Shortly before his hospitalization he had become homeless, living in his pickup truck for 5 days, looking at the bridge, and considering suicide while still spending $100–$200 a day in crack cocaine. He had not eaten for 3 days prior to admission. On the morning of his admission, he took 12 ibuprofen tablets and smoked more crack in an attempt to kill himself. Instead, he fell asleep for almost the whole day. That night, he made his way to the bridge determined to jump.

After the Highway Patrol picked him up and brought him to the hospital, he was initially evaluated for overdose. Toxicology tests demonstrated evidence of cocaine in his urine. He had lost 8–10 pounds in a 3-week period, had no appetite, and had been sleeping a couple of hours in the early mornings. He showed marked anhedonia, expressed guilt because of his drug abuse, and denied intentions of killing himself but stated he needed help with his crack abuse problem. After 3 days in a psychiatric emergency unit, he was admitted to a Black Focus inpatient and substance abuse program. During the admission process, he appeared anxious and tearful. He continued to demonstrate depressed mood, and, in view of his recent suicide attempts, he was placed under special surveillance.

Past Psychiatric History

Mr. D stated that he had been depressed since the death of his father 5 years ago. When he had learned of his father's death, he immediately left for Kenya. He drank heavily on the plane and arrived during the funeral proceedings. He was to give the traditional eulogy, which was his duty as the only son. Instead he stated, "I saw my dad's body there and passed out. I didn't attend the service." At the gravesite he was the first to be called to shovel the dirt, but he again became upset and was taken away. He stated that his wife called every day asking for his return: "I could have stayed a lot longer and taken care of business, but instead I got into a lot of trouble by getting drunk in clubs and becoming violent." He got into fights in bars with people. His family felt embarrassed and regarded him as a "disgrace." He states that they put him on a plane back to the United States to protect themselves from further embarrassment. Consequently, he stated that he was unable to "say a formal good-bye" to his father and thereby fulfill the customary duties expected of a first-born son.

Back in the United States he had success in his business but still had great difficulties in dealing with his feelings about his father's death, which he identifies as a stressor leading also to his continuous drug abuse. The cycle returned, this time with the abuse of crystal methamphetamine. "I got high as soon as I got off the plane." He stated that he became so despondent that he "walked away from the Church." He started questioning God: "Why did this have to happen?" He wouldn't share his doubts with his wife because he regarded her as being "too religious."

When prodded, the patient reported that he had felt some sadness since childhood. However, he was "not supposed to show it," since according to his cultural norms men are strong and do not show emotions:

"You are supposed to persevere despite adversities." He related how four of his close school friends back in Kenya had committed suicide in their teens: two drank DIP (an industrial-strength agent that is used to kill parasites in cows), another was very unhappy and died under mysterious circumstances, and the fourth drove off a cliff with a tractor because his father had died.

General Medical History

Mr. D denied any history of major medical illness. He had never been hospitalized, and he specifically denied history of head trauma or any surgical procedure. He was traditionally circumcised at age 12 in a hospital setting. He had no history of seizure disorders. Mr. D had had BCG vaccination at the age of 4 in Kenya, and he denied any history of active TB.

History of Substance Abuse

The patient had abused alcohol dating back to when he was 12 years old. His father and uncles owned a lodge where there was liquor available. He and his friends would "empty the glasses" of alcohol left. As he grew older, he would drink a six-pack per day of a strong local beer. His goal in drinking was to pass out. His alcohol use declined after he began to use crystal methamphetamine in the United States. Unable to obtain the drug when the family moved to a major city, he began using $100–$200 worth of crack cocaine per day. He would often pick up a local woman, and he would smoke cocaine in the garage from about 2:00 to 5:00 P.M., stopping when his wife and children came home. He would carry out a pretense of being the family man until the children were in bed, then resume smoking crack in the garage. His wife would ask him to come to bed, but he would always delay until she was fast asleep. He denied IV use of drugs, and he had no history of HIV infection. He had never been in drug treatment.

Personal Psychosocial/Developmental History

Early Childhood

Mr. D was born in Kenya, the first child and only son of a businessman and politician father. His mother was deeply engaged in the family business. The family was described as wealthy, "not very traditional," and educated. The father managed a production and distribution company involving sugar, salt, beer and shoes. The family lived on a large farm complex that included five large homes (one for each of the uncles). He lived with his parents and four younger sisters until age 12. The patient had good interaction with his sisters. His fondest childhood memories consisted of taking his dogs and a backpack full of sandwiches and spending days along a nearby river. He dreamed of finding the source of the river, a dream he eventually turned into reality. Mr. D continued to enjoy swimming, fishing, and other outdoor activities he had cultivated as a boy.

Social/Occupational History

Religious principles were an important aspect of Mr. D's family life. He was raised as a Catholic, and he therefore claimed that his life had been deeply rooted in Catholic principles. Furthermore, the age-grade system practiced by the Kikuyu tribe determined the role each individual was expected to play. When he was 12, he was subjected to the traditional ritual of circumcision, which was, however, modified for him in that the operation took place in a nearby hospital. The rites of passage at initiation were characterized by a sequence of instruction, socialization, and behavior change as each participant assumed a new role (of man or maiden). He was required to undergo complete initiation into manhood by living in his own cabin away from the main house. He stated that he "hated" sleeping alone and away from the rest of the family. Eventually he started "hanging out" with some older boys who lived in the Catholic seminary dormitory. From these relationships he speaks about leading "a double life…there has always been a good and a bad part." On the one hand, he was a good student and an altar boy who taught catechism; on the other, he was a mischievous class clown who sneaked alcohol from the family home.

Mr. D attended a private school while growing up in Kenya. He reported that there was only one other black student, but he had no particularly outstanding memory from this experience. His scholastic performance was good. He graduated from high school and went on to a Jesuit college in Kenya, where he attended for several years but received no degree.

At the age of 17, Mr. D met his current wife. She was a 20-year-old white woman from an American midwestern city, who was in Kenya as a missionary and teacher. He described it as a "love at first sight" experience for both of them. His family at first considered the relationship "cute," but as time went on his mother became uncomfortable. His father, however, remained supportive. The girl's parents were also divided along the same lines: father supportive and mother opposed. The couple worked very hard at the relationship so that it would prevail. As the relationship evolved, Mr. D had to face a huge dilemma when he learned that his girlfriend had become pregnant. At first he denied this to his mother, but he later admitted the child was his. His mother was visibly distressed, but his father continued to be supportive, encouraged Mr. D, and insisted that he should "do the right thing and marry her." Mr. D felt that his mother's dreams of his becoming a priest had been in vain and that he had disappointed her greatly. He stated that if he had his way, he would still be single.

In fact, the couple did not marry until 2 years later. After the marriage, Mr. D reported that his wife wanted to move back to the United States because "she had friends here." He claimed that he found the United States "terrifying" and he felt homesick every day. His wife's friends were educated and successful; it was overwhelming for him to be around them.

He secured a job as installer of insulation materials in new houses. The couple had three children: the firstborn a son, who is now 10, and two daughters, ages 8 and 6.

Family History

The patient reported no history of psychiatric illnesses among the members of his large immediate family. As stated above, Mr. D considered the death of his father 5 years prior to admission to be the most tragic event in his life. He had not seen his father for at least 5 years, and, following a tribal custom, he had never been told of his father's illness (diabetes). The news of his father's death devastated him, particularly because he had felt closer to him than he did to his mother. Mr. D loved his mother but considered her cold, rigid, and almost intolerant about views different from hers. The patient's oldest sister was a nun working in Nigeria. The other sisters were all married and living in Kenya.

Physical Examination

On admission to the psychiatric unit, the examination revealed that the patient was a soft-spoken Kenyan male in no acute physical distress; height 5 feet 9 inches, weight 140 pounds. Vital signs were well within normal limits. He was alert and oriented. Physical examination was unremarkable. There was no evidence of track marks, and the abdomen was soft, with no obvious sequelae of his previous history of alcoholism.

Laboratory tests were normal except that urine was positive for cocaine, blood acetaminophen <4, and salicylate <10. Routine chest X ray was normal.

Mental Status Examination

The patient was a thin man looking his stated age, dressed casually in blue jeans most of the time. He was cooperative, very polite, and friendly. He tended to use humor as a defense mechanism against painful feelings. There was no psychomotor agitation; rather, psychomotor retardation was noticeable. His mood was depressed, and he had sagging facial features with some evidence of frowning at the brow. He complained of 3 weeks of neurovegetative signs such as insomnia, loss of appetite, and weight loss; likewise, he had difficulties in concentration, some memory problems, and feelings of guilt. He showed, however, a wide range of affect, from labile to occasional inappropriate laughter while discussing painful topics. At times he would express deep grief and become tearful. Frequently, he would relate his feelings of guilt to how much his mother needed him back in Africa to help manage his father's inheritance and the family's life. The patient continued to ventilate suicidal feelings as he expressed how devastated he was at the prospect of numerous losses. He kept on saying "I have hurt the people I love the most." He remained impulsive, with a high probability of hurting himself, but denied suicidal thoughts while in the unit. Mr. D showed no evidence of psychotic symptomatology: his thought processes appeared linear and goal directed. He expressed motivation to enter a drug abuse treatment program.

Diagnostic Tests

Neuropsychological testing when the patient was sober and during the hospitalization revealed a moderate to severe impairment on verbal memory tasks. Projective testing and clinical interviews showed a significant degree of depression. He tended to compartmentalize his feelings as an attempt to avoid negative affect. Tests also unveiled a number of issues related to personal identity, which led to his playing roles others expected, making it difficult for him to be aware of his real wants and desires.

DSM-IV-TR Diagnosis

Axis I

Cocaine dependence

Major depression, single episode, severe, without psychotic features

Cocaine-induced mood disorder

Cognitive disorder NOS

History of alcohol abuse

History of methamphetamine dependence

Religious or spiritual problem

Axis II

Deferred

Axis III

None

Axis IV

Psychosocial stressors: problems related to multiple losses (father's death, separation, alienation from family and country of origin) and associated drug abuse; continuous acculturation problems; homelessness; unemployment

Axis V

GAF at time of diagnosis=50; past year: unknown

Case Summary

Clearly, Mr. D's depressive symptomatology can be accounted for by numerous losses in his life. The one that stands out is the loss of his father 5 years prior to this episode. Such loss was enmeshed with the loss of his country through immigration to the United States. He had failed to maintain links with his family because of substance abuse; hence the presence of guilt feelings. In turn, substance abuse may have been a self-medicating attempt, which only intensified guilt and loss of self-esteem. He did not realize that drugs cause depression, thus creating a vicious circle. Things got worse because his mother, as well as the rest of the family, needed him to play important roles as prescribed by the Kikuyu tribe— roles he was unable to fulfill. He tended to use denial as a defense mechanism generated by his growing up in a cultural environment where it was not proper for males to demonstrate feelings. He intellectualized and used humor to downplay hurtful feelings. Similarly, rationalization emerged whenever he discussed issues about his wife, whom he regarded as a "religious fanatic," making this an excuse for keeping his substance abuse a secret from her. He realized that his wife, a devout Catholic, would not accept such behavior. Identity issues play a vital role, as he claimed that there "is a good part and also a bad part in my life."

Differential Diagnosis

The possibility of a dysthymic disorder could not be dismissed, even though his overall functioning was apparently normal for many years. Chronic bereavement might have evolved into major depression, aggravated by his substance abuse. The duration factor argued against the possibility of an adjustment disorder. Anxiety features were not relevant, and posttraumatic stress disorder, dissociated somatization, or medical disorders that might have accounted for his main symptoms were absent. Personality features, without reaching the disorder level, could include passive-aggressive, avoidant, and dependent ones.

Cultural Formulation

Cultural Identity of the Individual

Mr. D was born and raised in Kenya, and he described himself as a Kenyan of the Kikuyu tribe. What was foremost in his identity was that he was black and African. He was aware of his upper-middle-class status in his native country, as evidenced by his continually reiterating that his family was considered wealthy and prosperous. The image of his deceased father and the influence he had wielded in the community earned Mr. D a special status as heir to a well-known family. His religious affiliation was also considered an important factor in his cultural identity. This man grew up as an altar boy serving in the local parish in a deeply devout Catholic family that instilled the principles of the Catholic faith deeply in his mind. He was a catechism instructor in the church. Throughout his stay in the hospital he commented that he had led a "double life," since his religious beliefs were in conflict with drug abuse and drinking alcohol.

We can infer that his identity as an African was complicated by the conflict between colonialism and allegiance to tribal and traditional beliefs. Furthermore, as an immigrant to the United States and throughout all his years in this country, he went through various phases of adjustment and restructuring of his life. Acculturation to the dominant culture was one of the severe stressors in his life. Since he was married to a white woman while maintaining his predominant African cultural identity, he became alienated from other African American persons and institutions. This issue may have been further complicated because his children are biracial and may not be accepted by his Kikuyu tribe. Mr. D grew up speaking Kikuyu; he also speaks Swahili. English was to him a second or third language. He remained ever conscious of his African accent as people asked, "Where is that accent from?"

Cultural Explanations of the Individual's Illness

The patient had several explanations for his illness. The first and foremost was built around his religious upbringing and Catholic faith. He was brought up with the belief that as long as you maintain a positive relationship with your Creator, everything in your life will go smoothly. In addition to his guilt-ridden "double life," Mr. D claimed that following the unexpected death of his father, he started having doubts about God's existence. He said he had many questions as he experienced a loss of faith. He attributed his substance abuse and current psychiatric symptomatology to this prevailing conflict. He regarded his depression as punishment for having challenged the principles which had been, for years, the pillars of his life. Stemming from this explanatory model, the treatment pathway included confession with a priest. There is no doubt that he manifested the features of a religious or spiritual problem, which needed appropriate intervention by a spiritual counselor or priest.

His second explanation was the inadequate mourning for his father. He felt that he had been unable to emerge from the grieving period because he did not have an opportunity to formally say good-bye to his father. Culturally, from the African and especially the Kikuyu tribe perspective, he was unable to fulfill the duties of the eldest son and heir by failing to assume a leadership role in the affairs of the family.

The third and very important explanation was his being outcast from the family because of alcohol abuse. As stated earlier, this man drank heavily during the time of his father's death. This had increased his guilt and low self-esteem. He expressed feelings of being ashamed for disrespecting his dead father.

Cultural Factors Related to Psychosocial Environment and Levels of Functioning

Mr. D suffered from many psychosocial stressors. Religion played a major part in his life as a source of both strength and stress. As mentioned earlier, the death of his father and the patient's subsequent response caused a significant degree of doubt and alienation from the Church and his family, whose rigid beliefs prevented closeness. At the same time he distanced himself from his wife and would not dare to discuss his doubts with her, much less win her support. He concealed his feelings and also felt inadequate to discuss the cocaine abuse problem. The wife was so religiously committed that he feared they would not communicate at the same level. Yet Mr. D still used the Church as a reference point in his life, since he continued to go for confession. It was through confession and the priest's advice that he was encouraged to "tell everything" about his drug abuse. The confession to his wife did not repair the breach, however, but further compromised the relationship, resulting in her leaving him and the house.

The family in Kenya, especially his father, had been a tremendous source of strength throughout his growing years, and the loss of his father was a major catastrophe in his life. His main internal conflict had to do with his shame and loss of esteem within his family and the Kikuyu tribe.

Finally, Mr. D grew up in a predominantly black environment, and interracial marriages were unknown or, at best, infrequent. The expectations of his culture were that he should marry within the Kikuyu tribe and bring up his children in its traditions. These expectations was stronger because he was the firstborn son of the family. Another important feature is that his wife was his former teacher while she worked in the Catholic mission. Thus, she remained the decision maker, a strong and dominant character, whereas Mr. D had always assumed a submissive role. Soon after getting married in Kenya, she insisted on moving to the United States. According to African culture, it is unusual for the man to follow the wife.

Cultural Elements of the Relationship Between the Individual and the Clinician

Mr. D was admitted to a special program unit (See Clinical Course, below). This was a unique feature in the case, because it facilitated an early development of positive rapport between the patient and the multidisciplinary treatment team. The patient was greeted with a high degree of empathy and was assured that he would be safe in the unit. His African accent was respectfully regarded and accepted. He met a team that was committed to the issues of diversity and to working with people of African descent. The psychiatrist was black, with extensive experience in treating black patients. The social worker connected immediately with Mr. D because of her cross-cultural experience; she had worked with professionals and patients from various parts of Africa. Mr. D also readily developed rapport with the occupational therapist as he was challenged with tasks that were reminiscent of those in African culture. The degree of empathy demonstrated by the team helped to promote the therapeutic alliance. He regarded the multidisciplinary team as the "Council of Elders," typical of African tradition, where all matters in the community were raised for solution.

Overall Cultural Assessment for Diagnosis and Care

The biopsychosocio-cultural-spiritual model was used. The cultural sensitivity of the treatment team facilitated the inclusion of the diagnostic category of religious or spiritual problem in the diagnosis. For appropriate intervention the patient needed to reconnect with the Church and use the priest to help resolve the conflict he was faced with. In the treatment planning, the patient's strengths—which included educational background, work history, and rich cultural heritage—were identified. After identification of the target symptoms and problems, the team developed a treatment plan to address the following dimensions:

- Biological: Substance abuse treatment, use of antidepressants (SSRIs).
- Psychological: Brief insight-oriented psychotherapy as well as supportive therapy, which used the information in the DSM-IV-TR Outline for Cultural Formulation. Grief counseling was used during the case conference.
- Socio-cultural: Involvement of the patient in various group activities, including Narcotics Anonymous and Alcoholics Anonymous. Culturally relevant occupational activities were used, such as engaging him in expressions of African art and African cooking. Ongoing efforts were made to engage his wife and children.
- Spiritual: Provision of support and appropriate referral to a chaplain or priest. The spiritual issues in the cultural context played a vital role in the resolution of grief.

Clinical Course

The initial hospital course was characterized by fluctuating episodes of depression and suicidality linked to developments occurring outside. On about day 7 of his hospitalization he stated, "I gave up the keys to my truck today so that my wife can sell it to pay for the needs of the children." His wife had told all his customers that he was no longer in business and sold his truck. He also lost his business contracts because he failed to keep his appointments. The patient was despondent about his situation, stating, "My life is over."

Furthermore, he initially objected to a treatment plan that would include his wife. He felt that his wife was "dominant" and that he often had to accede to her wishes. Periodically he would show outbursts of anger, lamenting that he was being punished by his wife: "I think she would like to see me on a street corner with a sign saying 'Will work for food.'" However, he missed his children very much, and he was further disturbed when he heard that his wife had moved to another neighborhood and had obtained a restraining order against him. One weekend, anger manifested itself as he broke the window in the unit right after the visit of his wife and children.

Mr. D started to take sertraline, 50 mg each morning, and the dose was increased to twice a day. On about day 13, sertraline was increased to 100 mg bid. As his insomnia continued, he was subsequently started on imipramine, 75 mg each day at bedtime; on day 19, the dose was increased to 150 mg until day 30, when the dose was increased to 200 mg each day at bedtime. The response was initially encouraging as the patient started having adequate sleep. His suicidal thoughts remained pervasive, however. The patient claimed he was not satisfied with imipramine and requested an alternative medication. He was started on trazodone, 50 mg each day at bedtime, later raised to 200 mg each day at bedtime; at this dose he started having more than 6 hours of sleep, and his depressive symptoms were also improving.

The major turning point during his hospitalization was reached when the multidisciplinary treatment team decided to convene a case conference on day 15. The unit in which he was treated follows the tenets of client-directed therapy. The patient was invited to be part of the case conference so that he could be actively involved in his care. Each team member presented his or her perspective on the case, and the patient interacted with the team. The team explored all the cultural issues involved, and Mr. D responded with powerful emotion, as evidenced by sobbing in response to descriptions of his shame and guilt. He was even more touched when it dawned on him that he had not fulfilled some of the necessary rituals following his father's death. Mr. D felt inadequate that he had not even placed the headstone at the father's grave since his death 5 years earlier. The patient expressed then his desire to return to Kenya so that he might complete the rituals necessary for the resolution of the grieving process. He expressed guilt again and said he was unable to face the thought of languishing in this country, abusing drugs, while his mother needed his support. At the end of the case conference, Mr. D felt comforted because the conference reminded him of the Council of Elders in his native Kenya. He had connected easily with this process and felt the treatment team's degree of support in his predicament.

On day 17 his status was changed from involuntary to voluntary. He started participating actively in groups, sharing his insights, and display-ing empathy for others. His occupational therapist continued to work with him by encouraging projects that were syntonic with his African cul-ture—for instance, during cooking groups he was encouraged to share with his peers some of the staple dishes from his country.

The patient was also involved in family therapy by the social worker, but, despite attempts to encourage couples' therapy, he systematically re-fused to join with his wife and the team. He said "I would like to entertain the option of couples' therapy after I have completed my recovery and I am back on my feet." It was difficult to determine the reasons for the pa-tient's resistance to couples' therapy. Perhaps this was a concept not in keeping with his culture, where gender roles are distinct and only close family members, not strangers, are involved in trying to resolve marital conflicts. His wife, however, had expressed her willingness to participate in couples' therapy.

The social worker as well as the multidisciplinary treatment team tried to look for a dual-diagnosis program that would meet the patient's needs after discharge. Eventually he was accepted into one that, although aware of the nature of the case, was mostly focused on homosexual HIV-positive persons. Not unexpectedly, Mr. D said that he didn't like the pro-gram. He says he was one of two people who were not gay and one of three who were not HIV positive. For him to be immersed in such a pro-gram was culturally dystonic, considering his cultural background, where homosexuality would not be a subject for discussion and was highly stig-matized. Despite all these barriers he felt that he should complete his sub-stance abuse treatment. He left after 2 months, and was in remission to the time of this writing.

There was significant improvement in the marital relationship as he and his wife were reunited. He said he had had a brief course of couples' therapy as well as a "special blessing ceremony" for their house conducted by a priest. He called this ceremony "enthronement," and the couple needed to make preparations for it several weeks in advance. It was obvious that religion or spirituality remained a strong point of reference in his life.

The follow-up interviews for more than a year after discharge showed that there had been progress since he had left the hospital. He reported that he was now gainfully employed at a sporting goods store as assistant manager. He was also enrolled in college part time. He continued to say that his involvement with the treatment team in the Black Focus Program had brought awareness to his life.

Discussion

This case study would be incomplete without looking into the cultural milieu in which the patient grew up. The East African Kikuyu-speaking tribe is one of the major groups that have been studied extensively. The Kikuyu arrived in Kenya about 1500 and were part of the migratory pattern that started in the Sahara region. They were middle-level agriculturalists whose main crops were maize and beans. They also kept goats, sheep, and a few cattle, which were more important for ritual than for dietary purposes. It was not uncommon for this tribe to join forces with others against a common enemy, despite the intermittent intratribal warfare for land control (Abbott 1976; Worthman and Whiting 1987).

The patient mentioned the roles that everyone played in his culture. According to the literature, a system of stratification based on age-grade existed for all individuals from childhood to old age (Mitchell and Abbott 1987; Worthman and Whiting 1987). The gradation ranged from childhood to elderhood for each gender. The males, for instance, were involved in military affairs early on in life, and the females played a major role in raising and preparing food, as well as taking care of the next generation. The sequence of age-grade for males was childhood; junior, then senior, warriorhood; junior, senior, and ritual elderhood. For females the sequence was similar, comprising childhood, maidenhood, young womanhood, junior elderhood, and elderhood. From this stratification we can see the importance of elderhood as the final stage in the development and growth of the individual. It is not surprising to see Mr. D aligning himself with the multidisciplinary team he regarded as a Council of Elders: female elders among the Kikuyu played a vital part in arranging and overseeing rituals and ceremonial activities. Political and judicial decisions were made by the junior and senior male elders. Ritual elders were responsible for performing the most sacred rites and ceremonies (Worthman and Whiting 1987).

The patient participated in the initiation according to Kikuyu tribal customs. The age-grade system played an essential role in defining adolescent life. The initiation took place early before puberty for girls and just after for boys. The initiation rite was marked by both physical and ritual components. The elaborate ceremony culminated in the genital operation for both sexes. The operation consisted of the excision of the tip of the clitoris for girls and slitting of the prepuce for boys. According to the tribal beliefs, the clitoris and prepuce were masculine and feminine body parts, respectively, and the operations were thus undertaken to correct or align the gender of the initiates. Initiation was followed by a sequence of instructions, socialization, and behavior change associated with the assumption of new roles as warriors and maidens. After the healing of the wounds the males had to undergo training as warriors, which lasted 9 years. The initiated girls entered maidenhood, which lasted until they were married. During this period they were expected to help their mothers with the work of adult women. One of the important outcomes of initiation was sexual education, which was conducted in the form of a lovemaking dance *(ngweko)* by the bachelors and young maidens. This dance was performed in a social gathering according to prescribed rules. The young maidens were instructed early on regarding techniques for avoiding genital contact. The culture does not allow discussion of sexual matters between parents and children (Worthman and Whiting 1987).

Kenya was a stronghold of British imperialism. Although colonialism imposes Western ideology, the pervasive traditional practices and beliefs remain predominant, which makes the individual straddle two worlds. Conflicts between traditional practices and acceptance of the practices of the colonial masters during the colonial period centered on land and female circumcision. The acquisition of land by the British made the Kikuyu warriors serve no function. The introduction of Christianity initiated a move to abolish female circumcision. With the introduction of education and further sophistication, circumcision had to be performed in hospital settings, as was the case with Mr. D. There is no doubt that social change had affected his adolescent experience, especially in matters of sex education. It is not surprising that Mr. D's relationship with his newly acquired girlfriend led to premarital pregnancy. Furthermore, a critical component of the case is the inordinate pressures of acculturation and the clashes (some of them unresolved) generated in the process. Some deserve mention: exposure to drug use and abuse, guardedness and secretiveness in the face of personal failures or of pressure to express deep-seated emotions, gender-role reversal with Mr. D's subjection to a strong female character (his wife), guilt related to notions bordering on betrayal of family of origin, and further alienation.

Depression among rural Kikuyu has been a subject of study by several investigators (Abbott and Klein 1979; Binitie 1975; Mitchell and Abbott 1987; Ndetei and Muhangi 1979). Females have higher rates of depression than males. Phillips and Segal (1969) suggested that women report more symptoms than men, based on cultural norms. Men are expected to be less expressive than women and hence hide their emotions (Mitchell and Abbott 1987). According to Prince (1968), who reviewed the literature regarding depression in Africans between 1890 and 1965, there is less verbalization of affect, less self-blame, and more projection of blame among men than among women. Agitation, anger, and excitement are some of the characteristics of African male depression that can often cause the depression itself to be missed or that can distort the diagnosis. Suicide appears to be rare. Intracultural variations in depression are characterized by the fact that acculturated Africans present in the Western manner, but unacculturated Africans do not. Somatic complaints seem to dominate; they may be complex and vary from abdominal complaints and headaches to creeping sensations under the skin and "worms" moving inside the head. On the whole, the manifestation of depression is culture bound and reflects community beliefs as well as communication styles (Binitie 1983). The complaints of bewitchment are a common feature even among the acculturated (Murphy 1979).

In this context, treatment, like the very existence of the Kikuyu, is built around rituals and ceremonies. As mentioned earlier, the raising of cattle, goats, and sheep in the economy of the Kikuyu was primarily for rituals. These rituals had a therapeutic effect on the lives of individuals. The sacrifice of animals was an important intervention in appeasing ancestors and restoring balance in the community (Binitie 1983). Because of the ritualistic manner of worship in Catholicism, it is not surprising that that religion was easily embraced by the tribe. For the same reasons, however, Mr. D's reluctance to move forward with needed interventions (such as couples' therapy or spiritual counseling), although understandable, represented a significant obstacle in his treatment, including early abandonment of treatment (even pharmacological). This also poses questions about his long-term prognosis, in spite of clear if tenuous improvement 1 year after discharge.

Finally, it is evident that since depression and anxiety are a feature of the Kikuyu and of African life, many cases may easily be missed in general practice unless the Western-trained clinician is aware of the uncommon manifestations of the disorder. Cultural competence plays a vital role in ensuring treatment compliance and successful outcome. More research is needed, however, to discover the part played by culture, spirituality, and rituals in facing transitions, acculturation problems, and full-fledged psychopathology, as well as in healing practices and outcomes.

■ References

Abbott S: Full-time farmers and weekend wives: an analysis of altering conjugal roles. Journal of Marriage and The Family 38:165–174, 1976

Abbott S, Klein R: Depression and anxiety among rural Kikuyu in Kenya. Ethos 7:161–188, 1979

Binitie A: A factor-analytical study of depression among cultures (African and European). Br J Psychiatry 127:559–563, 1975

Binitie A: The depressed and anxious patient: care and treatment in Africa. International Journal of Mental Health 12:44–57, 1983

DeVries MW, Sameroff AJ: Culture and temperament: influences on infant temperament in three East African societies, in Annual Progress in Child Psychiatry and Child Development. Edited by Chess S. New York, Brunner/Mazel, 1985, pp 191–202

Mitchell S, Abbott S: Gender and symptoms of depression and anxiety among Kikuyu secondary school students in Kenya. Social Science and Medicine 24:303–316, 1987

Murphy HB: Depression, witchcraft beliefs and super-ego development in preliterate societies. Canadian Journal of Psychiatry 24:437–449, 1979

Ndetei DM, Muhangi J: The prevalence and clinical presentation of psychiatric illness in a rural setting in Kenya. Br J Psychiatry 135:269–272, 1979

Phillips D, Segal B: Sexual status and psychiatric symptoms. American Sociological Review 34:58–62, 1969

Prince RH: The changing picture of depressive symptoms in Africa: is it fact or diagnostic fiction? Journal of African Studies 1:177–186, 1968

Worthman CM, Whiting JW: Social change in adolescent sexual behavior, mate selection, and premarital pregnancy rates in a Kikuyu community. Ethos 15:145–165, 1987

■ The "Good Catholic Girl"

Gender is related to a number of disorders. Women often present with complaints of being "anxious and depressed," and in many instances this is an idiom to signal feelings of demoralization and low self-esteem. Clinical experience in the treatment of women in American society suggests that this problem often results from disruptions in relationships with men. It is important to understand this idiom of distress and its sociocultural significance in the lives and psychology of women. This case study focuses on gender, age, and religion as cultural variables in complex interplay with developmental issues, personality organization, and symptom development while illustrating the importance of idioms of distress in psychiatric diagnosis and treatment.

Identifying Data

Ms. E was a 30-year-old, single, white female, the oldest of four children. She described herself as "predominantly" Irish American, from a middle-class Catholic background. At time of coming for treatment, she was completing graduate school in sociology and working part time in a shelter for homeless women.

Reason for Evaluation

Ms. E complained of feeling "anxious and depressed" since the breakup of a relationship with a boyfriend 6 months ago. Since that time she had felt desperate, unable to function, and convinced that she will never have a fulfilling relationship with a man. She said she needed a "lifeline."

History of Present Illness

Ms. E reported that she had been "depressed, sad, and irritable for most of her life." Since adolescence, she had felt unsure of herself, pessimistic, and somewhat hopeless. She had seen no need to seek treatment until this time because she had been able to function by putting forth a little extra effort.

Involved with Mr. F for 2 years, she had often questioned whether he was a good choice. He was not interested in pursuing his education, moved from one low-level job to another, and appeared to have no long-term goals. At times he seemed unsupportive and threatened by her ambition and success. She convinced herself these issues were not very important and that she and Mr. F wold eventually get married. During the last 6 months of their relationship, however, Mr. F began to withdraw from her and she discovered that he was having an affair.

Since the breakup with Mr. F, Ms. E had felt unable to function and had struggled to complete her academic work. She felt sad but denied any major changes in her appetite or sleep and said she still enjoyed doing things with her friends on occasion and sometimes felt OK. Feelings of guilt were always a part of her Catholic upbringing, but they seemed no worse than usual at this time. She felt hopeless about her relationships with men, but she had not thought of death or suicide.

Past Psychiatric History

Following her brother's death, 10 years ago, she had seen a counselor with her family for a brief period of time.

General Medical History

Ms. E reported that she had had all the usual childhood illnesses, but she denied any major medical illness, physical trauma, or surgery. She had stopped taking birth control pills a few years ago, and she was not on any prescribed medications. She had had her annual physical examination 6 months before coming for treatment, and her doctor told her that she was in good health. She exercised regularly and felt well physically.

Ms. E denied any past abuse or current use of drugs. She had never smoked cigarettes. She occasionally had a glass of wine with dinner when out with friends.

Developmental History

Throughout childhood, Ms. E felt constrained and inhibited. She felt incompetent, socially awkward, and on the outside of her peer group. She had few friends and was never allowed to sleep over or go places with the other children. She spent most of her time studying and going to church. She said she now felt angry and in conflict with her overprotective mother, who she believed caused her to be inhibited and ill prepared for womanhood.

After graduating from high school, she welcomed the opportunity to leave home and to go to college in order to prove that she was self-sufficient and independent. She worked part time and put herself through school. She studied hard and was successful academically, became involved in many extracurricular activities, and developed many friend-ships, but she still felt constrained and unsure of herself. After completing college, she worked for several years, then applied to graduate school to pursue a Ph.D.

Ms. E had had a series of relationships with men beginning in the eleventh grade. The first relationship seemed idyllic, but it ended soon after she left home for college. In college, she dated casually and had sev-eral short relationships, in which she felt devoted and helpful to the men but emotionally distant. She became sexually active in college, but she was tense and guarded and never experienced the degree of pleasure that she had expected. Mr. F was her first serious, long-term relationship. Despite some problems, she had been committed and determined and had felt certain that this relationship would "go the distance" and lead to marriage.

Social History

Ms. E lived alone in her own apartment, something she took pride in. Be-ing independent and able to take care of herself and manage her life had always been important to her. Despite long-term relationships with a few friends, she at times felt at a distance from them emotionally. Ms. E's mother still had a difficult time conveying her confidence in her, and Ms. E felt she had to remind her mother that she was a mature adult woman and could manage herself in the world.

Occupational History

Ms. E worked to put herself through college with jobs in service-related areas. She was going to school full time, pursuing a Ph.D. in sociology. She also volunteered in a homeless shelter for women, which she felt gave her the opportunity to help women become more resourceful and better able to manage their lives.

Family History

Ms. E described her mother as an "anxious, depressed and pessimistic woman who probably needed treatment." Ms. E's mother was very de-pendent on her own mother, who lived with the family. Ms. E remem-bered her mother's being overprotective and critical of her, always complaining and never satisfied. She was an intimidating, guilt-invoking Catholic disciplinarian.

Ms. E described her father as a hard-working self-employed insurance salesman devoted to providing for the family. He focused his attentions on his children and seemed to be controlled by their mother. Ms. E had a close relationship with her father and tried to please him. He took special pride and pleasure in her achievements. Her father had developed hypertension several years before the time of this case, but was otherwise in good health.

Ms. E was the oldest of four children. A brother four years younger (the older of the two brothers) was killed by a drunk driver at the age of 16. The family was in counseling for a brief period following the brother's death, but there is no formal history of psychiatric illness or psychiatric problems in the extended family. A younger sister, 25 years old and recently married, worked as a librarian. A younger brother, 23 years old, was in his first year of medical school. Ms. E recalled feeling envious of the older of her two younger brothers, who seemed to have more freedom and privilege than she. She perceived her younger sister and brother to be more indulged. Yet she felt special in her role as the eldest child and attempted to distinguish herself through her academic achievements.

Ms. E's maternal grandmother lived with the family until she died of complications of heart disease when Ms. E was 13 years old. Ms. E remembers her grandmother with warm, fond feelings.

Review of Systems

The review of systems revealed no major complaints.

Physical Examination

A physical examination shortly before she came for treatment revealed no evidence of abnormalities on clinical examination or laboratory studies.

Mental Status Examination

Ms. E was a tall, attractive, demure, slightly overweight young white woman. She wore glasses and dressed very conservatively. She was sad, anxious, and preoccupied with feelings of incompetence and helplessness. She reported that she felt distracted and unable to concentrate and was obsessively preoccupied. Ms. E complained of feeling "out of touch" with herself, with no sense of her true emotions. She reported that she had experienced a lot of hurt and disappointment in her life. At times she felt very angry, but she had no way to express it. She was always trying to please others in order to be accepted. Frequently she felt self-conscious, shameful, and humiliated over insignificant things. She was stalled and inhibited in life, afraid to make independent decisions and hesitant to move forward. She was never quite satisfied with the results of her efforts and was overly concerned about others' responses. At times she felt a bit hopeless, as if nothing was worth the effort. She denied, however, any suicidal ideation, plan, or intent.

Throughout the interview Ms. E tracked the therapist's facial expressions and posture as if she were fearful of being scrutinized, judged, and found wanting. She was overly concerned about doing things right (or doing things as she anticipated the therapist would expect of her), and she frequently solicited reassurance. She wanted to understand what was going on with her and to find better ways to manage her feelings.

Diagnostic Tests

Routine blood tests, including thyroid function tests, were within normal limits.

DSM-IV-TR Diagnosis

Axis I
Dysthymic disorder
R/O bereavement, complicated
R/O major depressive episode

Axis II
Personality disorder NOS, with dependent and obsessive-compulsive features

Axis III
None

Axis IV
Disruption of relationship; academic problem

Axis V
GAF=70 (current)

Differential Diagnosis

Ms. E presented with history of a chronic mood disorder, manifested by dysphoria, irritability, low energy, poor self-esteem, and feelings of hopelessness. Her mood had more often been low than not (since adolescence) and without swings, elevation, or expansive feelings. Since the breakup of the relationship with her boyfriend 6 months previously, she had been more "anxious and depressed," with decreased productivity and secondarily with academic problems.

Because the mood disorder had been chronic, persistent, and of mild to moderate severity since adolescence, it met criteria for dysthymic disorder. Although Ms. E described herself as more "anxious and depressed" and had had some difficulty functioning since the breakup of her relationship, she also acknowledged that she usually functions at a higher level than she subjectively feels capable of. A period of bereavement would have been expected after the loss of the relationship. There is a history of two major losses during the course of her life: the death of her grandmother when she was 13 years old and the traumatic death of her brother when she was 20 years old. There is some likelihood that the mourning process was not completed with regard to these losses. She felt tremendous envy and ambivalence toward the older brother who died. In the context of these issues, bereavement could be prolonged or complicated or could precipitate a secondary major depressive episode.

Her recent difficulties, precipitated by the breakup with her boyfriend, appeared to be an intensification of her usual depressive state. These symptoms, however, were of limited severity, lacked major vegetative symptoms, were associated with substantial conflict, and did not meet criteria for a major depressive episode.

Cultural Formulation

Cultural Identity of the Individual

Neither she nor any of her immediate family members had been to Ireland, but they maintained some sense of identification with these ethnic roots. Otherwise she believed that she had a mainstream, white American, suburban upbringing.

However, the family had strong religious beliefs in Catholic doctrine and practices that guided their lives and behavior. Her mother was a strict disciplinarian and invoked guilt in a "Catholic way." Ms. E's sense of herself was that she was "a good Catholic girl."

Ms. E's identity as a woman was important in her overall sense of herself. She took pride in the fact that as a woman she was competent and self-sufficient. Yet she struggled to achieve what she had come to believe was the ultimate accomplishment of womanhood: marriage and a family.

Cultural Explanations of the Individual's Illness

Ms. E's predominant idiom of distress is that she was "anxious and depressed." Although this had been a chronic mood state, it was accentuated by the recent loss of a relationship with a man. This particular idiom of distress allowed her to deny the less culturally acceptable feelings of anger and rage unacceptable to her as a woman and a good Catholic.

In many cultures, it is acceptable for women, in comparison to men, to be weak, dependent, helpless, and devastated in the face of loss. This may cause others to minimize the severity of women's expression of symptoms. At the same time, women are more likely to seek mental health care for their emotional distress and to seek it more immediately.

Cultural Factors Related to Psychosocial Environment and
Levels of Functioning

Ms. E had always turned to men, as she had turned to her father in early childhood, to provide her sense of self-worth. As she moved into her thirties, developmental, psychological, and sociocultural influences converged, causing her to place superordinate value on the relationship with a man. She felt she should have a man so she could marry and have a baby. The loss of this relationship, even with a man about whom she had substantial doubts, undermined her sense of self and self-worth. Despite her competencies and achievements, she had trouble regulating her self-esteem in the absence of a relationship with a man. Ms. E's illness permitted her to acknowledge her dependency needs, allowed her to seek professional help, and mobilized her friends and family in her support. She could also turn to her religion as a source of comfort and to restore her sense of hope. She could now escape without guilt, for the time being, from the many role responsibilities and expectations that others had of her and that she had of herself.

Cultural Elements of the Relationship Between the
Individual and the Clinician

The match in the therapeutic dyad of this Irish American white patient with an African American female therapist provided a unique situation.

As a female, the therapist could more easily become both the object of transference and the model of identification. The patient had experienced her mother as weak, helpless, and overburdened, and Ms. E was identified with her. As an African American, the therapist was perceived by the patient as a competent and successful woman who had made it against the odds. This would challenge the patient and give her permission to acknowledge her own competency in the face of overcoming the obstacles of gender and racial/ethnic group. She could also feel safe that her anger would not destroy this "mother/therapist," who was perceived to be a strong black woman. She could rework unresolved oedipal issues, resolve her superego guilt, and gain access to the capacity for deeper emotions and the ability to experience more fully the pleasures of a relationship with a man.

Overall Cultural Assessment for Diagnosis and Care

Several cultural issues were relevant to accurate diagnosis and treatment in Ms. E's case. They included the following:

1. The importance of idioms of distress
2. The significance of relationships in female development
3. Sociocultural influences in defining role responsibilities and expectations of women
4. The role of Irish Catholicism in personality organization
5. The female's use of the male in the regulation of self-esteem
6. Adaptational tasks in female identity development
7. Age as a transitional nodal point in adult female development

Clinical Course

Ms. E was seen in twice-weekly individual psychoanalytically oriented psychotherapy. She was convinced that her troubles were deeper than the most recent event and was hopeful that long-term analytically oriented therapy would help her to resolve these deep-seated issues.

The early phase of treatment was dominated by issues of control, compliance, and trust. Ms. E was extremely anxious and preoccupied with her feelings of incompetence and helplessness. She feared the relationship with the therapist, convinced that she would be scrutinized, judged, and found wanting. She was concerned about doing things right, and she wanted to be a good and compliant patient. Any clarification or challenge of her perceptions was experienced as an assault meant to shame and punish her. She did not want to be challenged by the therapist, only soothed and reassured.

She approached therapy like a confessional, reporting her sins and her badness, in an intellectualized manner and with isolation of affect, in hopes of obtaining forgiveness. She described feeling like a "dead zomie," created things to worry about, warded off the arousal of her intense yearnings and repressed anger, and deprived herself of any sense of pleasure. She developed a sadomasochistically tinged maternal transference with herself in the role of martyr.

Continued interpretation of her martyr role—assumed to ward off anticipated injury by the therapist and at the same time to solicit maternal concern—gradually restored a sense of trust and safety in the therapeutic alliance. She became more affectively alive, felt connected, and began to trust that perhaps the therapist, a woman (but unlike her anxious, depressed mother) could ultimately help her to develop the capacity to regulate her tension states.

This shift in the therapy was preceded by the following dream: "I was picking away a thick layer of skin like plaster of Paris. Underneath was a layer that was pink and healthy. I was amused and entranced by it."

Thus she began to expose her deepest longings, her intense rage, and her spontaneous impulses. She mourned the loss of the relationship with Mr. F as well as the illusion of an ideal relationship that had never existed. She revisited the early relationship with her mother and her own feelings of helplessness and rage. She had abundant memories revealing her attempts to accommodate her mother's dysphoric moods while always feeling powerless to effect an empathic connection. Ms. E had experienced herself as a burden and her needs as insatiable. These feelings undermined her enthusiasm and excitement and interfered with the consolidation of a sense of herself and her potentialities.

Throughout the treatment it was necessary to observe for the patient her constriction and inhibitions, compelled by her internalized perceptions of what was becoming of a woman, particularly a "good Catholic girl." This gradually led to an increasing sense of comfort in 1) taking pride in herself, 2) self-assertion, and 3) more prompt and direct expression of angry feelings and competitive strivings. Gradually she was able to relinquish the perception of herself as the incompetent, helpless child. She began to move out of her masochistic position and became less compliant and more insistent on the legitimacy of her needs.

As a result of the treatment, the patient acquired an increasing capacity to integrate and regulate her tensions and mood states and moved beyond her previous constrictions and inhibitions. She gained insight into her previous choice of men and her interactions with them as influenced by her early experiences and her unreal expectations and fears. Over time, she developed a stable, mature relationship with a man quite different from her previous selection, a man who was less easily maternalized. In this relationship she became freer in her affective expression and the level of pleasure she allowed herself to experience. She no longer felt the need to be such a good Catholic girl. She developed a level of maturity in her feminine development that allowed her to acknowledge both her strivings and her competencies. Similarly, she began to experience her ambition and achievement with a sense of deliberateness and purposefulness. She was able to take pride in these activities, gaining a more balanced sense and experience of her self-worth.

Discussion

From a psychodynamic perspective, it is clear that the patient had a difficult time establishing trust and that there were restrictions in her affective expression in relationships, especially with men. She had trouble with the recognition, acknowledgment, and expression of both her libidinal yearnings and her anger. Repression of these affects resulted in an experience of emotional deadness or inability to connect with others. Because of her emotional aloofness, either she selected men who were similarly emotionally aloof, or her relationships with men failed to develop the degree of emotional investment necessary for sustaining an enduring commitment. Ultimately she would be left feeling unlovable and powerless to effect a caring, empathic response and investment from others. The patient harbored resentment toward her mother for what she experienced as her mother's emotional unavailability and her difficulties in helping Ms. E learn to feel confident in herself. She believed that this left her ill prepared for womanhood. Because of her rage and ambivalence toward her mother, she was unable to successfully work through issues of separation, autonomy, and identity with her mother. Ms. E's anxiety about separation and loss was further intensified as a result of the death of her grandmother during her adolescence. Her maternal grandmother was an important self object, providing empathy and affirmation for Ms. E during the early stages of her development. Her grandmother's death was a significant loss and occurred at a critical stage of her development (age 13), during the time when the patient was beginning the second separation-individuation process in an attempt to solidify her identification and to move forward developmentally.

The patient was overly compliant and had a tendency to subordinate her needs. This behavior had its origins in her earlier experiences of her mother's empathic failures. Her mother was a depressed, anxious, preoccupied woman. This caused the patient, in her interactions with her mother, to perceive herself as a difficult, greedy child who overburdened her mother and who was unlovable. She defended against her frustration and rage by developing a sadomasochistically tinged relationship with her mother. As long as she was compliant, she felt assured that she would have access to whatever her mother was emotionally able or willing to give her (Chodorow 1978; Stoller 1968).

The patient, through her academic achievements, secondarily turned to her father. She performed for him and solicited his positive mirroring and maternal nurturance. Thus the man became for her both the forbidden oedipal object whom she sought to seduce and the holder of the power to provide her with a sense of self-worth. At the same time, she felt much ambivalence and anger toward men, originating in her rivalrous sibling relationship with her deceased brother. The brother was the first son, the "privileged, golden-haired boy," a threat whom she feared would rob her of her favored position as the eldest child. This fear was often acted out and further encumbered her relationships with men.

Although these are general issues for women, there may be different emphasis across cultures and depending on family background or socioeconomic status. African American women, although empathic to the plight of their male counterparts, are encouraged and given permission to be independent and self-sufficient. Asian and Indian women may be bound to their culture's expectation of their respect for and subservience to the man's authoritarian role. Hispanic women may sustain their male partners' machismo to compensate for their struggles and to maintain family harmony. On the other hand, white women who perceive their counterparts as powerful may be more likely to accommodate in hopes of sharing that power. It should be kept in mind, however, that there is much diversity within ethnic groups and that individual women choose differently how to cope and to function, in ways that either empower or disempower themselves (Comas-Diaz and Greene 1994).

Ms. E's Catholic upbringing was a significant element in her attitudes about herself and her defensive patterns, as well as influencing how she related to the therapist and her approach to the therapeutic process. The role that religion plays in the organization and sense of self, behavior, and interactions with others is a complex process (Lukoff et al. 1992). The degree of internalization (Ryan et al. 1993) or functional practice of religious beliefs may vary. Religion as a cultural factor, however, plays a significant role in mental health (Jensen et al. 1993). It influences defensive organization and the management of emotions, self-esteem regulation, the experience of well-being, and psychological integration and adaptation.

In a study of a group of Roman Catholic patients, Keddy et al. (1990) identified a tendency toward intellectualized orientation and problems in handling emotions. Clinical experience with women patients, even from moderately devout Catholic families, reveals how they struggle with feelings of guilt and inhibition, especially in the experience and expression of sexuality and of angry feelings. In the therapeutic situation, it is as if they offer a mea culpa to the therapist, searching for absolution and for permission to take full charge of their emotional senses. The religious identification, life, and sense of spirituality (regardless of the negative or positive role it plays in the lives of patients) cannot be disregarded in treatment. Keddy et al. (1990) suggested the need for treatment interventions to emphasize emotional integration for these patients. Leavy (1988) stated the case for psychoanalysis, finding no contradiction between analysis and faith. He suggested that the work of the analyst is to bring suffering persons closer to their true nature, purified of neurotic conflicts, narcissistic impediments, and developmental failures, in order that they may become more fully human and authentically themselves.

The normal developmental challenges that Ms. E was confronted with during adolescence could not be successfully negotiated in the context of earlier conflicts and the inability, at that stage, to comfortably use her mother as a model for identification. The major adaptational task for the adolescent girl, as for the adult woman throughout the life cycle, is the process of separation-individuation, and with it the establishment of a sense of herself—her personal and feminine role identifications apart from her mother—in the fulfillment of womanhood (Bland 1994). The sociocultural contributions to this struggle (as well as the role of mother and father) and its progressive and regressive shifts cannot be underestimated. These shifts are more apparent in the face of transitional nodal points—for example, graduation, first job or apartment, initiation or breakup of relationships. Society and culture define, restrict, and offer contradictory messages that create substantial conflict for girls as they attempt to reconcile the sense of their personal and their feminine self, to discover acceptable role identifications, and to maintain their self-esteem.

To be effective in the treatment of girls and women, the clinician must additionally be aware of these cultural influences and their interface with individual or internalized conflicts; and the clinician must also be able to guide young women through this struggle as they attempt to navigate a world that disregards, restricts, and gives contradictory messages about their femaleness. The ultimate task for women in treatment as they work through their individual conflicts is to internalize a confident inner sense of self and to actualize their potentialities in diverse roles, competencies, and loving relationships.

■ References

Bland IJ: Adolescent girl to woman: developmental issues in transition. Louisiana Psychiatric Association Newsletter 29:1–2, Winter 1994

Chodorow N: The Reproduction of Mothering: Psychoanalysis and the Sociology of Gender. Berkeley, CA, University of California Press, 1978

Comas-Diaz L, Greene B: Women of Color: Integrating Ethnic and Gender Identities in Psychotherapy. New York, Guilford, 1994

Jensen LC, Jensen J, Wiederhold T: Religiosity, denomination, and mental health among young men and women. Psychol Rep 72:1157–1158, 1993

Keddy PJ, Erdberg P, Sammon SD: The psychological assessment of Catholic clergy and religious leaders referred for residential treatment. Pastoral Psychology 38:147–159, 1990

Leavy SA: In the Image of God: A Psychoanalyst's View. New Haven, CT, Yale University Press, 1988

Lukoff D, Lu F, Turner R: Toward a more culturally sensitive DSM-IV: psycho religious and psychospiritual problems. J Nerv Ment Dis 180:673–82, 1992

Ryan RM, Rigby S, King K: Two types of religious internalization and their relations to religious orientations and mental health. J Pers Soc Psychol 65:586–96, 1993

Stoller RJ: The sense of femaleness. Psychoanal Q 37:42–55, 1968

■ A South American Minister

This case discusses the existential, interpersonal, and clinical experiences of an immigrant Protestant minister from Ecuador, a predominantly Catholic South American country. Coming to the United States as pastor of a Hispanic church in a predominantly white small town affected his adaptation and his family's life, perspectives, and expectations and resulted in his chronic depression. The patient's religious background provided a continuous sounding board for his experience in therapy. Enhancement of his self-esteem through a visit to his country of origin in the midst of the psychotherapeutic process contributed to a positive outcome.

Identifying Data

Mr. G was a 56-year-old Baptist church pastor in a midsize city of the southeastern United States. Born in Ecuador, he was the oldest of four children. At the time of coming to treatment, he had been married for 29 years and was the father of four. An immigrant in the United States since the early 1980s, he came in summer 1994 to a university-based outpatient clinic, referred by his oldest daughter, a master's degree candidate in sociology at an out-of-state university. He had specifically requested a Spanish-speaking therapist in order to "communicate better" his and his family's concerns.

Reason for Evaluation

The patient complained of feeling "very depressed" for several months, which he attributed to worries about H, his 24-year-old daughter, who had been diagnosed with diabetes 8 years previously and had married a 31-year-old Central American man whom the patient considered "irresponsible."

History of Present Illness

The patient reported feeling very "frustrated, depressed, impotent to change the course of events" for months, perhaps even years. Mr. G felt that he had "lost control" on a few occasions, very much against his style of "trying to be calm and objective, since trying to help other people is my duty." In addition to his increased depressive symptoms, he felt that he could not perform intellectually at the same level he had been accustomed to: "I have lost interest, energy, enthusiasm. I cannot concentrate."

He was worried that his relationship with his wife had been deteriorating over the last few years and reported that he and his wife were barely speaking to each other and that he felt neglected, abandoned, even ignored. He complained that the sexual aspect of their relationship was "practically down to nothing." He stated that he had felt forced to masturbate and was empty, frustrated, and guilty because his wife was so cold and unresponsive. He said that in the present period of turmoil "my sexual instincts have increased, and I have no outlet for that." He worried about his oldest daughter, who had been raped about a year before he came to treatment. He was distressed and asked, "Why did I come to this country? What am I doing here?" He complained about language problems, about his hard work with his church and charity organizations, and about the cultural conflicts of being in a foreign country; he said that all his efforts to succeed were unrecognized by others.

He felt that his ability to "fight depression" was being consistently eroded. He denied any suicidal ideation but admitted feeling increasingly tired and "in need of rest." He also complained of irregular sleep, occasional headaches, and reduced appetite, although he had not experienced weight loss. He felt reluctant to talk about his problems with another person, and he had never seen a psychiatrist before, "because I always thought I could solve my problems with God's help."

Past Psychiatric History

Mr. G had no recollection of previous "depressions," but his report suggested mild affective symptoms for years. He had never considered seeking professional help before.

General Medical History

Apart from the usual childhood diseases, he denied ailments. Since the beginning of the recent difficulties, he had been experiencing myalgias, occasional headaches, and "heartburn" that had required the occasional use of drugstore antacids. He had not visited a physician's office in the 4 years before coming for treatment.

History of Substance Abuse

Mr. G said he drank alcohol only on social occasions and did not smoke. He denied any drug use.

Personal History

Mr. G was the oldest of eight children born in a small rural town in Ecuador. He remembered the overwhelming poverty surrounding him and his family during his childhood: scarcity of food, long absences by his father going away to find work in the fields, and the frequent crying of his siblings. His father was a hardworking, quiet, religious man. His mother was also quiet and was devoted to her children and her husband. He remembers her gathering the children twice a day to pray together. He remembers being a serious and studious boy who loved to read "everything I could" as soon as he taught himself to do so. When he was 10, his father moved the family to a piece of land over the banks of the biggest river in the region, which "my father spotted, and so we started from scratch." For the next 4 years he worked hard helping his father in his new surroundings. He felt close to his father then. His father brought in a young cousin to help with the work. He remembers that this cousin also taught him to masturbate and gave him a Bible, which he started reading avidly. He felt called to a religious vocation then, although it did not materialize until late adolescence. He also spoke about being fondled by one of his father's farm workers between the ages of 12 and 15 ("he used to do it every morning"). He remembered feeling guilt and shame but also feeling excited, and he would go looking for the man who would "suck from my penis."

He started school at the age of 14 and was a distinguished student. He used to observe how others were playful, gregarious, and capable of engaging in group activities, and he regretted not being like them. He had his first girlfriend at the age of 15 in the school, and they engaged in heavy petting but no intercourse. At the age of 19 he moved to a large city on his own in order to further his education. He says that leaving his family was not a traumatic event, because he felt ready to go on with his life. He first took mail-order courses toward a teaching degree, but he then enrolled in a Bible institute, where he became acquainted with some Baptist ministers from the United States who were starting their missionary work in the area. He was inspired by their message (he had grown up in a traditional Catholic family) and their work and made up his mind then to become a minister. He gradually became prominent in this small Protestant group in the context of a predominantly Catholic community. The relationship with his family remained cordial, but was strained because of his conversion to a Protestant religion.

In the period between finishing his clerical studies and starting a job in a local church, he met a young woman from the Bible institute. She was, in Mr. G's words, "quite attractive and very popular." Nevertheless, because of his shyness, they barely talked. However, after a relationship lasting 8 years, they had been married 29 years before he came for treatment.

Occupational History

After spending 6 years in Quito, the capital city, he returned to his town in 1978, first as coordinator of religious studies in the Bible institute, where he later became director. He started reading texts in English and, although not fluent, was able to communicate with visiting ministers from the United States, who invited him to the church headquarters in Indianapolis in 1979. He finally persuaded his wife, and in 1981 they decided to leave their country and come to the United States.

His first assignment was in a community of farm workers of Mexican origin, in a very poor section of the city, many of them unable to speak English and shunned by the predominant Anglo community. A few years later, he moved to a larger community where he held a job for the 7 years prior to treatment. Mr. G gained there a degree of visibility in the community, which he seemed to enjoy. He worked hard, had a radio show once a week, taught, preached, related to other churches in the community, and sometimes found himself in the role of social mediator. He felt the pressures of a growing conflict between the Hispanic and African American communities in his town. He seemed to be both bothered and puzzled by these developments, had been forced to intervene at times, and felt that the situation might get worse. He did not talk too much about his own feelings as a representative of a minority in a predominantly white community, except to say that "the relationships between Hispanics and whites are better than between Hispanics and blacks."

Family History

The patient was unable to give detailed information about his eight siblings and parents. His said that two of his siblings had been married and then separated (he emphasized that divorce "is not allowed by the Church") and that one "may have had some problem with alcohol" but that that apparently had been resolved. Mr. G was not aware of any history of psychiatric diagnosis in his family.

The patient's 52-year-old wife seemed to have shown some behavioral changes over the years. She was reluctant to come to the United States, and more recently, with all the family turmoil, she was insisting that they go back. She had grown increasingly bitter, resentful, distant, and critical. More recently, he said, she had been moody, with pessimistic thoughts and hopelessness. Mr. G occasionally worries about her having a "touch of Alzheimer's." She had recently lost weight. Nevertheless, Ms. G had refused professional help.

His story of his four children revealed ambivalent feelings, negative emotions, frustrations, shattered dreams, self-reproach, anger, and many-faceted criticisms. When the family decided to come to the United States, his oldest son was looking forward to studying to be a doctor in Ecuador. He opposed the migration to the United States, and after they came, he decided to become a paramedic instead. He had a 2-year-old illegitimate child who lived with his mother in a northeastern city. Mr. G wonders about what could have happened had they decided to stay in their native country.

His second son was a musician, married to an American girl, and apparently doing relatively well. Again, Mr. G felt that this son, being as bright as his older brother, should have worked toward a professional degree. With both of his sons, his level of communication appeared to be quite limited: they called home from time to time, but not often, and apparently did not have much to talk about when they did.

His oldest daughter was a master's degree candidate in sociology in New York, and after the trauma of being raped, was doing well and planned to be married soon. Nevertheless, Mr. G ruminated about her behavior, which "went against all our moral principles and she caused me a great deal of pain." He said that she had lived with a man against all religious and moral beliefs. She had numerous boyfriends and did not pay any attention to what her parents were telling her. Finally, the youngest daughter, H, suffered from diabetes but was a strong character, and she loved her husband, who Mr. G felt was a quiet, cold, sometimes even rude individual who had become frustrated with his wife's illness. H confessed to her mother that around the age of 6 or 7 years she was sexually molested and that it had been in her mind all the time. At her worst, her weight was 67 pounds; at the time of this case, she was around 100 pounds but losing weight rapidly. H had been in and out of hospitals in recent months, much to Mr. G's frustration, consternation, and constant worry, "I listen to her whenever she tries to cry. I encourage her to do so, but I don't talk too much—I even appear to be indifferent—but, in reality, I suffer a lot."

Physical Examination

Vital signs were all within normal limits. Review of systems and a general physical examination were normal.

Mental Status Examination

Mr. G was a well-developed, well-nourished, soft-spoken, polite, overtly formal man who looked slightly younger than his stated age. He was dark skinned and of short stature, appropriately dressed, well oriented to time, place, and person. He showed relatively poor eye contact yet was cooperative and apparently willing to discuss the most relevant issues of his condition. His speech was regular in rate and rhythm, his voice inflections somewhat monotonous but in general appropriate. He looked tense, particularly when talking about his daughter H's condition and the difficult times that he and his family were going through; he also voiced depressive feelings and symptoms, such as poor concentration, occasional apathy, a tendency to isolate himself, increasing irritability, helplessness, and occasional physical symptoms such as fatigue and headaches. Nevertheless, he denied suicidal or homicidal ideation. He smiled enigmatically at times, particularly when responding to questions on specific family-related matters or personal reactions. His answers were almost always cautious and guarded. He seemed to have doubts about some of them, pondering the questions and his responses in a somewhat obsessive way, but without reaching a clinical dimension. There was no evidence of psychosis. His judgment seemed to be appropriate, and his insight appeared to be fair.

Functional Assessment and Diagnostic Tests

The patient seemed to be functioning appropriately in his everyday life activities (see DSM-IV-TR axes IV and V below), even though pressures and strains were noticeable. The Mini-Mental State Exam was normal, with a score of 28/30. Additional psychological and diagnostic tests were not deemed necessary.

DSM-IV-TR Diagnosis

Axis I
Dysthymia
R/O generalized anxiety disorder
R/O major depression

Axis II

Passive-aggressive, schizoid/avoidant, obsessive-compulsive, and narcissistic personality features

Axis III

History of probably gastroesophageal reflux disorder (GERD)

Axis IV

Daughter's health problems
Marital difficulties
Wife's behavioral and emotional changes
Work pressures and demands
Issues of cultural identity, acculturation, and perception by others

Axis V

GAF=65

Chronic low-grade depression seemed to have marked this patient's everyday behavior, overlapping with prominent Axis II features such as interpersonal insecurity, overcontrolling impulses, tendency to isolate himself, hypersensitivity, self-doubts, and desire to impress others. He was resentful for perceived lack of recognition by his peers, members of his church, and his family. He also exhibited excessive self-control and efforts to avoid overt expression of emotions.

Moreover, the patient's depression was centered on the stresses in important areas of his life. The failures of some of his children in his eyes and the illness of his daughter were narcissistic wounds that made him feel self-critical and made him direct anger toward himself.

Cultural Formulation

Cultural Identity of the Individual

Mr. G was a Hispanic immigrant from Ecuador with only a fair degree of acculturation to United States society. Born and raised as Catholic, he became a Protestant minister as a young adult. His parishioners were Spanish-speaking people of limited education and therefore themselves alienated from the host culture. It became obvious that he and his wife as well as their children spoke Spanish at home, he watched mostly Spanish-language television channels, and he specifically sought to talk about his problems in Spanish.

Cultural Explanations of the Individual's Illness

Mr. G said his problems were related to his suffering for his daughter's brittle physical condition. He found ready support for these explanatory models from his wife and perhaps his children, all of them possibly intent on trying to minimize and/or deny the meaning of intrafamily conflicts and having culturally related differing philosophies. Another explanatory level was his thinking that his problems were a test of his religious strength and fortitude. He also saw the problems as the work of the "enemy" (Satan), while insisting on the support he derived from his faith. He prayed continuously and asked for God's help in his situation. This religious self-support appeared to be only partially protecting him from the disharmony within the family.

Cultural Factors Related to Psychosocial Environment and
Levels of Functioning

Mr. G followed a religious career as a way to get out of the social stratum in which he and his family of origin were embedded. He used his intellectual talents, reading interests, and knowledge of the Bible as a way to move ahead, subtly mixing such circumstances with his natural tendency to be shy, private, submissive, and quiet in order to impress others. He moved to the United States, thinking it would exalt his social status, found himself a member of the Hispanic minority in a West Coast suburban town, and worked as a pastor in a Protestant church (a minority church among Hispanics) in two cities where Hispanics were also a deprived minority. In other words, he exhibited three levels of a pervasive minority status: ethnic, social, and religious.

In addition, the role of religion may have been overplayed, without any effective sign of support during the patient's ordeal. The degree of family support appeared to be minimal; he extracted some social support from the church activities but found himself doing so in his role of pastor—that is, taking care of others without necessarily being taken care of himself. Other than his nuclear family, he had no other relatives in this country, and apparently his family ties in his country of origin were also significantly reduced. He sensed that his accomplishments also appeared to be minimized, misunderstood, or ignored. He found solace in reading his Bible, other religious books and newspapers, and watching TV news and shows, preferably in Spanish. As a compensatory maneuver he idealized everything in his native country, unwittingly contributing to his own sense of alienation. Furthermore, he felt that one of the main reasons for his coming to the United States was that "I wanted my children to have better education and opportunities." The cultural shock, plus the barriers of language and his own pastoral obligations, made him feel frustrated, particularly because only one of their children has reached "a good academic level." His sons, even though employed, "have not been able to improve their lives." It should also be noted that his son-in-law, although also a Hispanic immigrant, came from a much poorer, more backward Central American country, and the son-in-law's difficulties might also have been increased by the obvious disrespect that Mr. G felt toward him.

Cultural Elements of the Relationship Between the Individual and the Clinician

Mr. G requested a Spanish-speaking therapist, which certainly put him at ease and provided him with a sense of being understood. Nevertheless, social status differences between the therapist (a psychiatrist) and the patient, as well as the traditional respect for the authority of the physician, posed some potential barriers; however, the patient did not voice any problems about the therapist and seemed to act comfortably in his presence. On the other hand, his excessive formality and shyness may have concealed his underlying feeling of social inferiority.

Overall Cultural Considerations

The ambivalence created by the experience of anger and frustration in an individual whose cultural identity put him in the special position of being targeted as an inferior minority was a constant source of distress and uncertainty. There were doubts and puzzlement in the patient's assessment of his own identity, his role within his family, and his job with a church community and with the population of the medium-sized city where he lived. This created uncertainties also about his adequacy as a husband and as a pastor. Self-esteem and self-image were based on the patient's identity and on his role in the community. They were also based on factors such as his premorbid personality, his work ethic, and his ambitions and expectations, all of which may have been dramatically shattered by coming to the United States, thus creating growing disillusionment, frustration, and ultimately clinical depression. His reluctance to seek professional help until the time he came for treatment was also culturally determined (shame, privacy, "sign of weakness," and the like). In addition, his family problems, the lack of support and understanding on the part of his wife, and the illness of his daughter were decisive contributing factors.

Clinical Course

Initial management consisted of sertraline, 150 mg qd, individual psycho-therapy, and couples' therapy. During the first several weeks, the thera-pist suggested that the patient write brief reports on events from his past that he considered relevant to what he was experiencing at the time of treatment. Thus, he discussed his early sexual experiences, the nature of his religious avocation, his illusions and expectations regarding his move to the United States, and his awareness about his wife's emotional condi-tion. However, he often focused on vague somatic complaints, on side effects of the medications (particularly those affecting his sexual perfor-mance), and on his daughters' physical or psychological problems. In fact, H was hospitalized at least twice a month during this initial phase of individual therapy. Interestingly enough, Mr. G continued demonstrating a rather tight self-control, never betraying any emotions, always smiling politely and trying to minimize the impact of intrafamily issues and events on his own psychological status. He always seemed very formal, used ra-tionalization, and considered his words carefully, trying in general to keep up a good front. Nevertheless, it was increasingly clear that a num-ber of undercurrents were governing the course of his therapy.

The three main areas of interest during this phase of therapy were family, marriage, and work. The first had been brought into sharp relief by the daughter's illness and her marriage to a man whom the patient considered inferior in every way (economically, socially, intellectually, culturally). He professed profound disregard for his son-in-law, whose history of substance abuse, lack of steady occupation, poor intellectual accomplishments, and lack of affection he criticized strongly. Mr. G was also critical of the career path followed by his oldest son, whom he had wanted to become a lawyer but who chose art and music instead. His fears of losing control of his family's fate were quite evident as the patient spoke of his responsibilities as a father, as a breadwinner, and as a role model for his children and his parishioners alike.

The patient soon related his concerns with his marriage. He largely glossed over their courtship period even though it lasted about 8 years; instead, he talked about the couple's strained interaction over the past several years, their temperamental differences, the roles they had played in the children's upbringing, and their different coping styles. His assessment of his wife and the marriage was critical. He complained that his wife tried to wrest from him control over their life as a couple, as well as running the family. She had criticized him continuously for his way of handling the children, to the point that he had decided "to remove myself from taking care of the kids." Consequently, he had let her assume control and devoted most of his energies to his ministry, his studies, his sermons, and his involvement with parishioners. She had stopped cooking for him and made continuous financial demands. The disagreements also reached the sexual arena and, to complicate matters even further, the couple had a very limited social life.

Another major problem for the patient was related to his work as a pastor. On several occasions he indicated that had he stayed in South America, "now I would be in a very big and high position in my church" and wondered whether coming to the United States "was worth the effort." He felt burdened by "having to deal with everybody else's problems, frustrations, and difficulties." At times he doubted the truth of his religious learnings, the existence of God, and the possibility of fairness and justice. He found it difficult at times to communicate in English and experienced anxiety and uncertainty about his role and his effectiveness.

It was clear that the patient was struggling with a tremendous amount of negative feelings, underlying anger, and a sense of frustration and impotence. He came closest to admitting this when talking about his confusion in the face of his wife's unpredictability. On occasions, he had found himself "reacting negatively, yelling at my wife, even hurting her." He has also found out that more recently "what used not to bother me, now hurts me. I am becoming more sensitive, more intolerant."

The patient's marital problems escalated, and it was decided to include Ms. G in the therapy. She was initially very reluctant to talk, complaining of depression, lack of concentration, easy fatigability, crying spells, restless sleep, lack of appetite, weight loss, lack of interest in her surroundings, and ideas of death. She also began taking sertraline and within the next 3 weeks felt better. Her improvement coincided with an improvement in their son-in-law's personal disposition toward them. At the same time Ms. G began talking more openly and directly about the nature of her relationship with Mr. G. She described him as quiet, noncommunicative, and selfish. She said that he preferred not being bothered: "he gets his newspaper or book and reads it even while watching television news." The wife remembered vividly how a few days after their wedding, she wanted to go out with him on Christmas Eve "just because I was so happy." He refused and went to bed at 9:00 P.M. The same thing happened during New Year's Eve, and Ms. G remembers herself "watching everybody being happy on the streets from the window of my apartment."

The patient's wife also spoke about the role of "victim" that Mr. G used to play in front of his children and in front of some other relatives whenever a disagreement between the two of them occurred. She said that he always described himself as being attacked and criticized when, in her opinion, he was rigid, intolerant, isolated, and "antisocial." She said that he always used work as "either an excuse or a refuge" and locked himself into his study. As a result, his level of communication with his children was as poor as it was with his wife. The word *machismo* was uttered many times during these therapy sessions. Mr. G, however, managed to present a good front, smiling continuously whenever his wife criticized him and patting her on the back in a condescending fashion.

The therapist's approach was to encourage increasing openness in the dialogue, making clear that this was not a confrontation but rather an effort to open up lines of communication between them. The therapist tried to deflate the intensity of the criticisms in order to preserve a degree of flexibility and negotiability between the two of them. Mr. G and his wife were encouraged to continue the dialogue at home, trying to find common ground, compromise, mutual acceptance, and a rediscovery of the positive roots of the relationship. Generally speaking, both appeared to be optimistic about the outcome.

After a 3-week visit to his native country, the patient returned "reinvigorated" by the warmth, respect, and admiration he had found among friends, relatives, and colleagues. Mr. G. began to talk about his pride in being able to extricate many families in his church from their interpersonal problems; on the other hand, he commented about the paradox of "being unable to solve my own domestic problems" but reaffirmed his trust in facing the future more successfully.

Discussion

Symptomatically, Mr. G had the significant somatic component seen in many Hispanics suffering from depression (Escobar et al. 1987; Magni et al. 1992). Furthermore, these somatic symptoms appeared to provide a good indicator of response to medication, prediction of clinical outcomes, and even the experiencing of predictable side effects. In other words, the symptoms improved as therapy progressed, and even when he had some relapses, the first indications were physical complaints (Shapiro 1995).

Mr. G had several additional cultural characteristics related to his age, status, occupation, and stage of marriage. He tried to exert control over a family that experienced much dissension. He was extremely guarded throughout the first phase of treatment, and he made clear that he had difficulties in trusting people. He harbored reservations about seeking professional help and protected his privacy and his particular life philosophy, but in contrast he also showed respect for formal authority. He also exhibited a desire to be praised, understood, supported, and recognized, characteristic of his Hispanic cultural background (Briones et al. 1990; Golding et al. 1991).

Religion also played an important role in this patient's story. It was an early anchor of identity, a defense against a hostile world, a ladder toward social improvement and recognition, a source of comfort and direction, and a rigid moral code that when violated caused a great deal of pain. His religious identity made him somehow special, making him stand apart from his fellow men, recognized by God. There is an extensive literature regarding the role of religion in Hispanic communities (Lukoff et al. 1995; Ruiz 1979). The rigid approach of many Hispanic heads of families makes them, on occasion, unable to deal with the different world views adopted by their children (Garza and Gallegos 1995).

Religion also played an important role in the explanatory approach of this patient to his clinical condition. He referred to the role of "the enemy" (Satan) in making his life miserable. Mr. G, however, was not the average religious Hispanic man, namely Catholic. He belonged to a Protestant denomination that, even though growing among the Latin American population, is still a minority and is looked upon with a sense of curiosity as well as hostility (González et al. 1995). Furthermore, he was a South American Hispanic immigrant, but, for the first several years of his ministry in the United States, he was dealing with a primarily Mexican American community composed of immigrants from Mexico or American-born Chicanos. Language and even racial or other culturally determined characteristics were not enough to forge a constructive link with his church members. It is clear that there are still significant differences between the various groups that are part of the Hispanic population of the United States (Puerto Ricans, Cubans, Mexican Americans, and Central and South Americans) (Lock 1993; Ring and Marquis 1991).

The many aspirations that have fallen short of full realization in an immigrant's life are sources of profound ambivalence, particularly among Hispanics, whose sense of pride, competitiveness, and hypersensitivity can make them susceptible to depressive psychopathology (Golding et al. 1991; Magni et al. 1992). Ambivalence stems from self-control, rigid moral principles, and respect for formalities, which prevent this group from openly expressing doubts, anger, self-commiseration, and rage. This constraint in turn makes symptoms worse and creates barriers in the psychotherapeutic process.

Mr. G was an idealistic man who became Baptist and came to the United States for "salvation": to achieve well-being, perfection, and grace. What he got instead was a series of challenging life problems: discrimination, rape, mediocrity, sickness, and the painful chronic illness and possible loss of a daughter. He was grieving the illusion of paradise lost, a sort of narcissistic redemption. He wanted to be extraordinary and became instead less than ordinary (Cortes 1994).

In spite of these apparently ingrained personality characteristics, psychotherapy appears to have produced some benefits. It was not only the shared language and other commonalities that contributed to this modest but sustained success. According to the patient, it was the possibility of trusting, opening up, and discussing personal issues without fear of being criticized, denounced, or stigmatized. He did not trust Hispanic ministers, much less American ministers, but he trusted a Spanish-speaking therapist once he made the decision to seek help. The therapeutic approach was based on a common cultural background but also on the reliance on reasoning abilities and the acceptance of realities in exchange for the reaffirmation of legitimate accomplishments and "good deeds"—concepts that are very close to the Hispanic collective persona (Escobar et al. 1987; Magni et al. 1992). The central issue of self-esteem in Mr. G's case was a crucial point in his therapy: a visit to his native country was a catalyzing experience, as he returned "rejuvenated" by the warmth, support, and admiration of his countrymen. This experience meant a great deal to him, and the halo effect of the visit lasted for a long period.

■ References

Briones DF, Heller PL, Chalfant HP, et al: Socioeconomic status, ethnicity, psychological distress and readiness to utilize a mental health facility. Am J Psychiatry 147:1333–1340, 1990

Cortes DH: Acculturation and its relevance to mental health, in Theoretical and Conceptual Issues in Hispanic Mental Health. Edited by Malgady RG, Rodriguez O. Malabar, FL, Krieger Publishing, 1994, pp 53–67

Escobar JI, Golding JM, Hough RL, et al: Somatization in the community: relationship to disability and use of services. Am J Public Health 77:837–840, 1987

Garza RT, Gallegos PI: Environmental influences and personal choice: a humanistic perspective on acculturation, in Hispanic Psychology. Edited by Padilla M. Thousand Oaks, CA, Sage, 1995, pp 3–14

Golding JM, Aneshensel CS, Hough RL: Responses to depression scale items among Mexican-Americans and non-Hispanic Whites. J Clin Psychol 47:61–75, 1991

González CA, Griffith EEH, Ruiz P: Cross-cultural issues in psychiatric treatment, in Treatments of Psychiatric Disorders, 2nd Edition, Vol 1. Edited by Gabbard GO. Washington, DC, American Psychiatric Press, 1995, pp 56–85

Lock P: The concept of race: An ideological construct. Transcultural Psychiatry Research Review 30:203–227, 1993

Lukoff D, Lu F, Turner R: Cultural considerations in the assessment and treatment of religious and spiritual problems. Psychiatr Clin North Am 18:467–486, 1995

Magni G, Rossi MR, Rigatti L, et al: Chronic abdominal pain and depression: epidemiological findings in the United States: Hispanic Health and Nutrition Examination Survey. Pain 49:77–85, 1992

Ring JM, Marquis P: Depression in a Latino immigrant medical population: an exploratory screening and diagnosis. Am J Orthopsychiatry 61:298–302, 1991

Ruiz P: Spiritism, mental health, and Puerto Ricans: an overview. Transcultural Psychiatry Research Review 16:28–43, 1979

Shapiro ER: Grief in family and cultural contexts: learning from Latino families. Cult Divers Ment Health 1:159–176, 1995

5

Conclusions

The overriding purpose of a book devoted to cultural assessment in clinical psychiatry is to emphasize the usefulness and practicality of cultural psychiatry's contributions to the everyday work of the clinician. Under the term *clinician* we include not only the psychiatrist subjected to a variety of complex theoretical orientations and clinical demands, but also all other mental health professionals working within multidisciplinary teams. Various cultural factors, different in intensity, duration, scope, and relationships with each other, constitute the background against which clinical events unfold. The cultural context, therefore, becomes not only a matter of descriptive value but also a crucial element influencing diagnosis, care planning, treatment, and prognosis.

■ A Historical Perspective

For cultural psychiatry to reach this level of clinical applicability, it had to make a sometimes stormy journey of historical developments. Much has happened from the time of the first comparative observations carried out in the late nineteenth century. At that time, European academicians surveyed non-European foreign cultures with a paternalistic eye and tried to establish diagnostic categories for them, which reflected only a limited understanding of their own transcultural efforts. Throughout the 1950s, psychodynamic principles enriched anthropological approaches to the

165

relationship between culture and personality, but these principles had limited clinical applicability. Today, a multidimensional contemporary perspective underlies specific diagnostic rules, clinical formulations, and policy recommendations thoroughly infused by cultural elements (Alarcón et al. 1999; Mezzich et al. 1996, 1999). Current treatment procedures recognize cultural variations at both the intrapersonal and the neurobiological levels. As a result (among other factors) of pressures from communities and the political body, the clinical value of culture in medicine and psychiatry is now more readily recognized. American pragmatism has prevailed over theoretical formulations, modern-day mythologies, and nonmedical considerations, resulting in improved diagnostic nomenclatures, delivery of care systems, and individual practices. In the process, cultural psychiatry has also redefined what it is and what it means, as well as what it is not and what it does not mean (Alarcón 1998). Ultimately, we hope this text has demonstrated that cultural psychiatry is more than a psychiatry of exotic syndromes or of ethnic minorities, a political tool, an antibiological school of thought, or simply "old wine in new bottles."

■ Cultural Variables

To understand culture and its effect on clinical events in psychiatric patients, the dissection of culture into its main variables seems to be a workable strategy. This entails the dynamic interaction of many areas of a person's life—his or her relation to

- The world
- His or her fellow human beings
- Society as the stage of interpersonal and personal/environmental interactions
- The areas of language, values, meanings, and history

At the same time, however, there is a sense of concreteness in the study and assessment of these variables as they are explored and evaluated in the clinical encounter.

There are different approaches to the grouping of these cultural variables. This book contemplates ethnicity, race, gender, and age as perhaps the most traditionally recognized. The first two, however, have always been controversial. Ethnicity represents the bedrock of personal identity (that perceived by oneself and others) in that it emphasizes identification with and belonging to a legacy, as well as integration with developmental processes (Johnson-Powell and Yamamoto 1997). At the same time, ethnicity entails internal variations that, although eroding assumptions of monolithic structures, reflect the rich weaving of diversity within well-identified groups. Race, as well, has become embroiled in considerable controversy and has been increasingly employed in political terminology (Carter 1995). Its use as a means of objective clarification is too often confused with the spelling out of values and attributes. However, it has been repeatedly proved that race is an invalid, unscientific parameter for the classification of human groups, because skin color and other physiognomic components vary immensely from group to group and even within groups (Comas-Diaz and Greene 1994). Yet race still plays an unjustified role in diagnostic and therapeutic practices in the United States. The factual and objective application of cultural psychiatry concepts will, it is hoped, overcome the unfair and subjective use of race as an element influencing patient–clinician interactions.

Gender, age, and education form a second set of variables in the study of culture. Epidemiological studies show that type and level of psychopathology vary as a function of gender, age, and level of education. Gender determines roles and behaviors born out of both understandable expectations and pervasive stereotypes (Comas-Diaz and Greene 1994; Young-Bruehl 1996). A notion linked to gender is, of course, that of sexual orientation, which has such an emotional impact on today's society, particularly as influenced by the emergence of groups such as homosexuals, bisexuals, and others who produce not only a unique set of views about mental health and mental illness in our society (Cabaj and Stein 1996) but also elicit responses from clinicians and the community at large that continuously reshape the fabric of contemporary culture. Age, as a concept closely related to developmental stages, creates at each level an array of culturally complex factors, not the least of which are those of stigma and subsequent neglect or mismanagement. Education also exerts crucial influence on the important cultural mechanism of acculturation.

In the United States and elsewhere, the subject of migration generates a heated debate. It has enormous clinical implications, regardless of the nature of the migration: spontaneous, forced, political, economic, internal, international, or intercontinental. Elements as varied as country of origin, socioeconomic status, and diet play a role uniquely fashioned by the migration experience. Diet, for instance, has both psychosocial and biological effects that undoubtedly affect the survival or demise of the individual and his or her group. Migrants bring with them myths, traditions, and beliefs that become both an anchor to the "old culture," a point of reference for the transactions with the host culture (acculturation), and either a helpful tool or an insurmountable barrier in the process of cultural assimilation. Needless to say, migration also defines the starting point on the socioeconomic ladder faced by the immigrant. All these interactions (acculturative stress) generate strong pathogenic, pathoplastic (the shaping and modalities of symptomatic expression), therapeutic, and diagnostic components in the assessment of any given patient.

Among the most important and complex cultural variables are religion and language. Religion and its nonorganizational variant, spirituality, influence the elaboration of explanatory models of illness as well as the therapeutic management of clinical conditions (Hood et al. 1996; Pargament 1997). Language, the best-understood means of communication among human groups, contains details and nuances that build the foundation for constructive interactions with clinicians, therapeutic teams, and the host culture; it can, however, also create significant obstacles to such relationships by planting the seeds of distortions and misunderstandings. Language also conveys symbolism, meaning, and perceptions of feelings such as warmth or hostility, affection or hatred, that are paramount human emotions (Good and Delvecchio-Good 1981).

It must be emphasized that culture does not entail denial or rejection of biological (specifically, neurobiological) factors in human behavior. Current research is capable of identifying the substrates of general, broadly defined emotions in a renewed effort to find a biological basis for what were once considered basically "subjective" phenomena. The universalistic, seemingly ruling trend of biological research should be balanced, however, by the notions that not every human action has a purely genetic basis, or that the nature-nurture, genetic-environmental, or biological-cultural polarities do include much between the opposites. It is the niche that Eisenberg (1998) or the interface that Hughes (1993) postulates as the crucial element of these interactive processes and that needs to be studied systematically and objectively. The answers are far from being tangible at this point, which should stimulate rather than deter future inquiry.

■ Implications for Training and Research

The pervasiveness of culture in everything that we do, think, or feel is undeniable in spite of some resistance among both the learned and the unsophisticated. Many issues of crucial impact on mental health are taking place the world over, creating more needs but also more opportunities. The disorientation of contemporary youth, the resurgence of ethnic identities, the polarization of hate and conflicts among nations old and new, and the rediscovery of religious fundamentalism are cultural phenomena that demand both deep studies and effective action. Culture—which also informs, whether we like it or not, the capacity and the effectiveness of political decision-making bodies—should be a critical element in these endeavors.

By adding a cultural dimension to the assessment process, the clinician expands the biopsychosocial approach to include conceptual and pragmatic subtleties that range from the ecological to the spiritual. The cultural approach adds to comprehensiveness of a case evaluation and expands both the clinician's understanding of the case and the patient's self-perception of his or her own suffering. The implications for education, training, and research are manifold.

The extraordinary advances of biological psychiatry can reach higher relevance only if an appropriate cultural view is rationally taught. The cultural component is an obligatory aspect of training for future psychiatrists and other mental health specialists and a required part of any certification process in the mental health professions. The future will see more of this deliberate effort at inclusiveness as demands in that direction keep coming from community and patient groups. The public will expect culturally competent systems of mental health care delivery as care providers realize that the use of health services is clearly contingent on offering truly comprehensive care. Conversely, payments will be denied if comprehensive care (which includes cultural issues) is overtly or covertly denied.

In the clinical research arena, culture has increasing relevance in general and specific fields. Among the former, outcomes research will be unable to ignore the role of culture in the study of procedures, tests, psychotherapeutic approaches, diagnostic criteria, and the newer area of disease management. By adjusting its methodology to the cultural characteristics of the patient groups under study, outcomes research will reflect the renewed emphasis on truly productive intervention techniques.

Finally, among specific research areas, the use of the components of the cultural formulation is a paramount topic, as is the possibility of creating measurement instruments for such components (Lewis-Fernández 1996). Similarly, cultural variables such as violence, race, age, and gender will attract increasing attention. This development is even more intriguing if we consider the increasing study of biocultural linkages, which it is hoped can explain in more detail the many mysteries of all mental disorders.

■ References

Alarcón RD (ed): Cultural Psychiatry. Psychiatr Clin North Am 18:449–465, 1995

Alarcón RD: What cultural psychiatry isn't. Psychline 2:27–28, 1998

Alarcón RD, Westermeyer J, Foulks EF, et al: Clinical Dimensions of Contemporary Cultural Psychiatry. J Nerv Ment Dis 187:465–471, 1999

Cabaj R, Stein T (eds): Textbook of Homosexuality and Mental Health. Washington, DC, American Psychiatric Press, 1996

Carter R: The Influence of Race and Racial Identity in Psychotherapy. New York, Wiley, 1995

Comas-Diaz L, Greene B (eds): Women of Color: Integrating Ethnic and Gender Identities in Psychotherapy. New York, Guilford, 1994

Eisenberg, L: The Harvey Shein Memorial Lecture, presented at 27th Annual Mid-Winter Meeting, American Association of Directors of Psychiatric Residency Training, Orlando, FL, January 17, 1998

Good B, Delvecchio-Good MJ: The meaning of symptoms: a cultural hermeneutic model for clinical practice, in The Relevance of Social Science for Medicine. Edited by Eisenberg L, Kleinman A. Dordrecht, Netherlands, Reidel, 1981, pp 165–196

Hood R, Spilka B, Hunsberger B, et al: The Psychology of Religion, 2nd Edition. New York, Guilford, 1996

Hughes R: Culture of Complaint: The Fraying of America. New York, Oxford University Press, 1993

Johnson-Powell G, Yamamoto J (eds): Transcultural Child Development: Psychological Assessment and Treatment. New York, Wiley, 1997

Lewis-Fernández R: Cultural formulation of psychiatric diagnosis. Cult Med Psychiatry 20:133–144, 1996

Mezzich JE, Kleinman A, Fabrega H, et al (eds): Culture and Psychiatric Diagnosis. Washington, DC, American Psychiatric Press, 1996

Mezzich JE, Kirmayer LJ, Kleinman A et al: The place of culture in DSM-IV. J Nerv Ment Dis 187: 457–464, 1999

Pargament K: The Psychology of Religion and Coping. New York, Guilford, 1997

Young-Bruehl E: The Anatomy of Prejudices. Cambridge, MA, Harvard University Press, 1996

GAP Publications

Cultural Assessment in Clinical Psychiatry (GAP Report 145, 2001), Formulated by the Committee on Cultural Psychiatry

Homosexuality and Mental Health: The Impact of Bias (GAP Report 144, 2000), Formulated by the Committee on Human Sexuality

In the Long Run...Longitudinal Studies of Psychopathology in Children (GAP Report 143, 1999), Formulated by the Committee on Child Psychiatry

Addiction Treatment: Avoiding Pitfalls—A Case Approach (GAP Report 142, 1998), Formulated by the Committee on Alcoholism and Addictions

Alcoholism in the United States: Racial and Ethnic Considerations (GAP Report 141, 1996), Formulated by the Committee on Cultural Psychiatry

Adolescent Suicide (GAP Report 140, 1996), Formulated by the Committee on Adolescence

Mental Health in Remote Rural Developing Areas: Concepts and Cases (GAP Report 139, 1995), Formulated by the Committee on Therapeutic Care

Introduction to Occupational Psychiatry (GAP Report 138, 1994), Formulated by the Committee on Occupational Psychiatry

Forced Into Treatment: The Role of Coercion in Clinical Practice (GAP Report 137, 1994), Formulated by the Committee on Government Policy

Resident's Guide to Treatment of People With Chronic Mental Illness (GAP Report 136, 1993), Formulated by the Committee on Psychiatry and the Community

Caring for People With Physical Impairment: The Journey Back (GAP Report 135, 1992), Formulated by the Committee on Handicaps

Beyond Symptom Suppression: Improving Long-Term Outcomes of Schizophrenia (GAP Report 134, 1992), Formulated by the Committee on Psychopathology

Psychotherapy in the Future (GAP Report 133, 1992), Formulated by the Committee on Therapy

Leaders and Followers: A Psychiatric Perspective on Religious Cults (GAP Report 132, 1992), Formulated by the Committee on Psychiatry and Religion

The Mental Health Professional and the Legal System (GAP Report 131, 1991), Formulated by the Committee on Psychiatry and the Law

Psychotherapy With College Students (GAP Report 130, 1990), Formulated by the Committee on the College Student

A Casebook in Psychiatric Ethics (GAP Report 129, 1990), Formulated by the Committee on Medical Education

Suicide and Ethnicity in the United States (GAP Report 128, 1989), Formulated by the Committee on Cultural Psychiatry

Psychiatric Prevention and the Family Life Cycle: Risk Reduction by Front-line Practitioners (GAP Report 127, 1989), Formulated by the Committee on Preventive Psychiatry

How Old Is Old Enough? The Ages of Rights and Responsibilities (GAP Report 126, 1989), Formulated by the Committee on Child Psychiatry

The Psychiatric Treatment of Alzheimer's Disease (GAP Report 125, 1988), Formulated by the Committee on Aging

Speaking Out for Psychiatry: A Handbook for Involvement With the Mass Media (GAP Report 124, 1987), Formulated by the Committee on Public Education

Us and Them: The Psychology of Ethnonationalism (GAP Report 123, 1987), Formulated by the Committee on International Relations

Psychiatry and Mental Health Professionals (GAP Report 122, 1987), Formulated by the Committee on Governmental Agencies

Interactive Fit: A Guide to Nonpsychotic Chronic Patients (GAP Report 121, 1987), Formulated by the Committee on Psychopathology

Teaching Psychotherapy in Contemporary Psychiatric Residency Training (GAP Report 120, 1986), Formulated by the Committee on Therapy

A Family Affair: Helping Families Cope With Mental Illness: A Guide for the Professions (GAP Report 119, 1986), Formulated by the Committee on Psychiatry and the Community

Crises of Adolescence—Teenage Pregnancy: Impact on Adolescent Development (GAP Report 118, 1986), Formulated by the Committee on Adolescence

The Family, the Patient, and the Psychiatric Hospital: Toward a New Model (GAP Report 117, 1985), Formulated by the Committee on Family

Research and the Complex Causality of the Schizophrenias (GAP Report 116, 1984), Formulated by the Committee on Research

Friends and Lovers in the College Years (GAP Report 115, 1983), Formulated by the Committee on the College Student

Mental Health and Aging: Approaches to Curriculum Development (GAP Report 114, 1983), Formulated by the Committee on Aging

Community Psychiatry: A Reappraisal (GAP Report 113, 1983), Formulated by the Committee on Psychiatry and the Community

The Child and Television Drama (GAP Report 112, 1982), Formulated by the Committee on Social Issues

The Process of Child Therapy (GAP Report 111, 1982), Formulated by the Committee on Child Psychiatry

The Positive Aspects of Long Term Hospitalization in the Public Sector for Chronic Psychiatric Patients (GAP Report 110, 1982), Formulated by the Committee on Psychopathology

Job Loss—A Psychiatric Perspective (GAP Report 109, 1982), Formulated by the Committee on Psychiatry in Industry

A Survival Manual for Medical Students (GAP Report 108, 1982), Formulated by the Committee on Medical Education

INTERFACES: A Communication Casebook for Mental Health Decision Makers (GAP Report 107, 1981), Formulated by the Committee on Mental Health Services

Divorce, Child Custody and the Family (GAP Report 106, 1980), Formulated by the Committee on Family

Mental Health and Primary Medical Care (GAP Report 105, 1980), Formulated by the Committee on Preventive Psychiatry

Psychiatric Consultation in Mental Retardation (GAP Report 104, 1979), Formulated by the Committee on Mental Retardation

Self-Involvement in the Middle East Conflict (GAP Report 103, 1978), Formulated by the Committee on International Relations

The Chronic Mental Patient in the Community (GAP Report 102, 1978), Formulated by the Committee on Psychiatry and the Community

Power and Authority in Adolescence: The Origins and Resolutions of Intergenerational Conflict (GAP Report 101, 1978), Formulated by the Committee on Adolescence

Psychotherapy and Its Financial Feasibility Within the National Health Care System (GAP Report 100, 1978), Formulated by the Committee on Therapy

What Price Compensation? (GAP Report 99, 1977), Formulated by the Committee on Psychiatry in Industry

Psychiatry and Sex Psychopath Legislation: The 30s to the 80s (GAP Report 98, 1977), Formulated by the Committee on Psychiatry and Law

Mysticism: Spiritual Quest or Psychic Disorder? (GAP Report 97, 1976), Formulated by the Committee on Psychiatry and Religion

Recertification: A Look at the Issues (GAP Report 96, 1976), Formulated by the Ad hoc Committee on Recertification

The Effect of the Method of Payment on Mental Health Care Practice (GAP Report 95, 1975), Formulated by the Committee on Governmental Agencies

The Psychiatrist and Public Welfare Agencies (GAP Report 94, 1975), Formulated by the Committee on Psychiatry and the Community

Pharmacotherapy and Psychotherapy: Paradoxes, Problems and Progress (GAP Report 93, 1975), Formulated by the Committee on Research

The Educated Woman: Prospects and Problems (GAP Report 92, 1975), Formulated by the Committee on the College Student

The Community Worker: A Response to Human Need (GAP Report 91, 1974), Formulated by the Committee on Therapeutic Care

Problems of Psychiatric Leadership (GAP Report 90, 1974), Formulated by the Committee on Therapy

Misuse of Psychiatry in the Criminal Courts: Competency to Stand Trial (GAP Report 89, 1974), Formulated by the Committee on Psychiatry and Law

Assessment of Sexual Function: A Guide to Interviewing (GAP Report 88, 1973), Formulated by the Committee on Medical Education

From Diagnosis to Treatment: An Approach to Treatment Planning for the Emotionally Disturbed Child (GAP Report 87, 1973), Formulated by the Committee on Child Psychiatry

Humane Reproduction (GAP Report 86, 1973), Formulated by the Committee on Preventive Psychiatry

The Welfare System and Mental Health (GAP Report 85, 1973), Formulated by the Committee on Psychiatry and Social Work

The Joys and Sorrows of Parenthood (GAP Report 84, 1973), Formulated by the Committee on Public Education

The VIP With Psychiatric Impairment (GAP Report 83, 1973), Formulated by the Committee on Governmental Agencies

Crisis in Child Mental Health: A Critical Assessment (GAP Report 82, 1972), Formulated by the Ad hoc Committee

The Aged and Community Mental Health: A Guide to Program Development (GAP Report 81, 1971), Formulated by the Committee on Aging

Drug Misuse: A Psychiatric View of a Modern Dilemma (GAP Report 80, 1970), Formulated by the Committee on Mental Health Services

Toward a Public Policy on Mental Health Care of the Elderly (GAP Report 79, 1970), Formulated by the Committee on Aging

The Field of Family Therapy (GAP Report 78, 1970), Formulated by the Committee on Family

Toward Therapeutic Care (2nd Edition—No. 51 revised) (GAP Report 77, 1970), Formulated by the Committee on Therapeutic Care

The Case History Method in the Study of Family Process (GAP Report 76, 1970), Formulated by the Committee on Family

The Right to Abortion: A Psychiatric View (GAP Report 75, 1969), Formulated by the Committee on Psychiatry and Law

The Psychiatrist and Public Issues (GAP Report 74, 1969), Formulated by the Committee on International Relations

Psychotherapy and the Dual Research Tradition (GAP Report 73, 1969), Formulated by the Committee on Therapy

Crisis in Psychiatric Hospitalization (GAP Report 72, 1969), Formulated by the Committee on Therapeutic Care

On Psychotherapy and Casework (GAP Report 71, 1969), Formulated by the Committee on Psychiatry and Social Work

The Nonpsychotic Alcoholic Patient and the Mental Hospital (GAP Report 70, 1968), Formulated by the Committee on Mental Health Services

The Dimensions of Community Psychiatry (GAP Report 69, 1968), Formulated by the Committee on Preventive Psychiatry

Normal Adolescence (GAP Report 68, 1968), Formulated by the Committee on Adolescence

The Psychic Function of Religion in Mental Illness and Health (GAP Report 67, 1968), Formulated by the Committee on Psychiatry and Religion

Mild Mental Retardation: A Growing Challenge to the Physician (GAP Report 66, 1967), Formulated by the Committee on Mental Retardation

The Recruitment and Training of the Research Psychiatrist (GAP Report 65, 1967), Formulated by the Committee on Psychopathology

Education for Community Psychiatry (GAP Report 64, 1967), Formulated by the Committee on Medical Education

Psychiatric Research and the Assessment of Change (GAP Report 63, 1966), Formulated by the Committee on Research

Psychopathological Disorders in Childhood: Theoretical Considerations and a Proposed Classification (GAP Report 62, 1966), Formulated by the Committee on Child Psychiatry

Laws Governing Hospitalization of the Mentally Ill (GAP Report 61, 1966), Formulated by the Committee on Psychiatry and Law

Sex and the College Student (GAP Report 60, 1965), Formulated by the Committee on the College Student

Psychiatry and the Aged: An Introductory Approach (GAP Report 59, 1965), Formulated by the Committee on Aging

Medical Practice and Psychiatry: The Impact of Changing Demands (GAP Report 58, 1964), Formulated by the Committee on Public Education

Psychiatric Aspects of the Prevention of Nuclear War (GAP Report 57, 1964), Formulated by the Committee on Social Issues

Mental Retardation: A Family Crisis—The Therapeutic Role of the Physician (GAP Report 56, 1963), Formulated by the Committee on Mental Retardation

Public Relations: A Responsibility of the Mental Hospital Administrator (GAP Report 55, 1963), Formulated by the Committee on Hospitals

The Preclinical Teaching of Psychiatry (GAP Report 54, 1962), Formulated by the Committee on Medical Education

Psychiatrists as Teachers in Schools of Social Work (GAP Report 53, 1962), Formulated by the Committee on Psychiatry and Social Work

The College Experience: A Focus for Psychiatric Research (GAP Report 52, 1962), Formulated by the Committee on the College Student

Toward Therapeutic Care: A Guide for Those Who Work With the Mentally Ill (GAP Report 51, 1961), Formulated by the Committee on Therapeutic Care

Problems of Estimating Changes in Frequency of Mental Disorders (GAP Report 50, 1961), Formulated by the Committee on Preventive Psychiatry

Reports in Psychotherapy: Initial Interviews (GAP Report 49, 1961), Formulated by the Committee on Therapy

Psychiatry and Religion: Some Steps Toward Mutual Understanding and Usefulness (GAP Report 48, 1960), Formulated by the Committee on Psychiatry and Religion

Preventive Psychiatry in the Armed Forces: With Some Implications for Civilian Use (GAP Report 47, 1960), Formulated by the Committee on Governmental Agencies

Administration of the Public Psychiatric Hospital (GAP Report 46, 1960), Formulated by the Committee on Hospitals

Confidentiality and Privileged Communication in the Practice of Psychiatry (GAP Report 45, 1960), Formulated by the Committee on Psychiatry and Law

The Psychiatrist and His Roles in a Mental Health Association (GAP Report 44, 1960), Formulated by the Committee on Public Education

Basic Considerations in Mental Retardation: A Preliminary Report (GAP Report 43, 1959), Formulated by the Committee on Mental Retardation

Some Observations on Controls in Psychiatric Research (GAP Report 42, 1959), Formulated by the Committee on Research

Working Abroad: A Discussion of Psychological Attitudes and Adaptation in New Situations (GAP Report 41, 1958), Formulated by the Committee on International Relations

Small Group Teaching in Psychiatry for Medical Students (GAP Report 40, 1958), Formulated by the Committee on Medical Education

The Psychiatrist's Interest in Leisure-Time Activities (GAP Report 39, 1958), Formulated by the Committee on Public Education

The Diagnostic Process in Child Psychiatry (GAP Report 38, 1958), Formulated by the Committee on Child Psychiatry

Emotional Aspects of School Desegregation (an abbreviated and less technical version of Report No. 37) (GAP Report 37A, 1960), Formulated by the Committee on Social Issues

Psychiatric Aspects of School Desegregation (GAP Report 37, 1957), Formulated by the Committee on Social Issues

The Person With Epilepsy at Work (GAP Report 36, 1957), Formulated by the Committee on Psychiatry in Industry

The Psychiatrist in Mental Health Education: Suggestions on Collaboration With Teachers (GAP Report 35, 1956), Formulated by the Committee on Public Education

The Consultant Psychiatrist in a Family Service Agency (GAP Report 34, 1956), Formulated by the Committee on Psychiatry and Social Work

Therapeutic Use of the Self (A Concept for Teaching Patient Care) (GAP Report 33, 1955), Formulated by the Committee on Psychiatric Nursing

Considerations on Personality Development in College Students (GAP Report 32, 1955), Formulated by the Committee on the College Student

Trends and Issues in Psychiatric Residency Programs (GAP Report 31, 1955), Formulated by the Committee on Medical Education

Report on Homosexuality With Particular Emphasis on This Problem in Governmental Agencies (GAP Report 30, 1955), Formulated by the Committee on Governmental Agencies

The Psychiatrist in Mental Health Education (GAP Report 29, 1954), Formulated by the Committee on Public Education

The Use of Psychiatrists in Government in Relation to International Problems (GAP Report 28, 1954), Formulated by the Committee on International Relations

Integration and Conflict in Family Behavior (Reissued in 1968 as No. 27A) (GAP Report 27, 1954), Formulated by the Committee on Family

Criminal Responsibility and Psychiatric Expert Testimony (GAP Report 26, 1954), Formulated by the Committee on Psychiatry and Law

Collaborative Research in Psychopathology (GAP Report 25, 1954), Formulated by the Committee on Psychopathology

Control and Treatment of Tuberculosis in Mental Hospitals (GAP Report 24, 1954), Formulated by the Committee on Hospitals

Outline to Be Used as a Guide to the Evaluation of Treatment in a Public Psychiatric Hospital (GAP Report 23, 1953), Formulated by the Committee on Hospitals

The Psychiatric Nurse in the Mental Hospital (GAP Report 22, 1952), Formulated by the Committee on Psychiatric Nursing—Committee on Hospitals

The Contribution of Child Psychiatry to Pediatric Training and Practice (GAP Report 21, 1952), Formulated by the Committee on Child Psychiatry

The Application of Psychiatry to Industry (GAP Report 20, 1951), Formulated by the Committee on Psychiatry in Industry

Introduction to the Psychiatric Aspects of Civil Defense (GAP Report 19, 1951), Formulated by the Committee on Governmental Agencies

Promotion of Mental Health in the Primary and Secondary Schools: An Evaluation of Four Projects (GAP Report 18, 1951), Formulated by the Committee on Preventive Psychiatry

The Role of Psychiatrists in Colleges and Universities (GAP Report 17, 1951), Formulated by the Committee on Academic Education

Psychiatric Social Work in the Psychiatric Clinic (GAP Report 16, 1950), Formulated by the Committee on Psychiatry and Social Work

Revised Electro-Shock Therapy Report (GAP Report 15, 1950), Formulated by the Committee on Therapy

The Problem of the Aged Patient in the Public Psychiatric Hospital (GAP Report 14, 1950), Formulated by the Committee on Hospitals

The Social Responsibility of Psychiatry: A Statement of Orientation (GAP Report 13, 1950), Formulated by the Committee on Social Issues

Basic Concepts in Child Psychiatry (GAP Report 12, 1950), Formulated by the Committee on Child Psychiatry

The Position of Psychiatrists in the Field of International Relations (GAP Report 11, 1950), Formulated by the Committee on International Relations

Psychiatrically Deviated Sex Offenders (GAP Report 10, 1950), Formulated by the Committee on Forensic Psychiatry

The Relation of Clinical Psychology to Psychiatry (GAP Report 9, 1949), Formulated by the Committee on Clinical Psychology

An Outline for Evaluation of a Community Program in Mental Hygiene (GAP Report 8, 1949), Formulated by the Committee on Cooperation With Lay Groups

Statistics Pertinent to Psychiatry in the United States (GAP Report 7, 1949), Formulated by the Committee on Hospitals

Research on Prefrontal Lobotomy (GAP Report 6, 1948), Formulated by the Committee on Research

Public Psychiatric Hospitals (GAP Report 5, 1948), Formulated by the Committee on Hospitals

Commitment Procedures (GAP Report 4, 1948), Formulated by the Committee on Forensic Psychiatry

Report on Medical Education (GAP Report 3, 1948), Formulated by the Committee on Medical Education

The Psychiatric Social Worker in the Psychiatric Hospital (GAP Report 2, 1948), Formulated by the Committee on Psychiatric Social Work

Shock Therapy (GAP Report 1, 1947), Formulated by the Committee on Therapy
Index to GAP Publications #1–#80

■ Symposia Reports

The Right to Die: Decision and Decision Makers (S-12, 1973), Formulated by the Committee on Aging

Death and Dying: Attitudes of Patient and Doctor (S-11, 1965), Formulated by the Committee on Aging

Urban America and the Planning of Mental Health Services (S-10, 1964), Formulated by the Committee on Preventive Psychiatry

Pavlovian Conditioning and American Psychiatry (S-9, 1964), Formulated by the Committee on Research

Medical Uses of Hypnosis (S-8, 1962), Formulated by the Committee on Medical Education

Application of Psychiatric Insights to Cross-Cultural Communication (S-7, 1961), Formulated by the Committee on International Relations

The Psychological and Medical Aspects of the Use of Nuclear Energy (S-6, 1960), Formulated by the Committee on Social Issues

Some Considerations of Early Attempts in Cooperation Between Religion and Psychiatry (S-5, 1958), Formulated by the Committee on Psychiatry and Religion

Methods of Forceful Indoctrination: Observations and Interviews (S-4, 1957), Formulated by the Committee on Social Issues

Factors Used to Increase the Susceptibility of Individuals to Forceful Indoctrination: Observations and Experiments (S-3, 1956), Formulated by the Committee on Social Issues

Illustrative Strategies for Research in Psychopathology in Mental Health (S-2, 1956), Formulated by the Committee on Psychopathology

Considerations Regarding the Loyalty Oath as a Manifestation of Current Social Tension and Anxiety (S-1, 1954), Formulated by the Committee on Social Issues

■ Films

Discussion Guide to the Film (2, 1970)
A Nice Kid Like You (1, 1970)

Index

Page numbers printed in **boldface** type refer to tables.

DATE DUE